sexualities in health and social care

a textbook

Tamsin Wilton

with cartoons by the author

Open University Press
Buckingham • Philadelphia

sexualities in health
and social care

**This book is to be returned on or before
the last date stamped b**

Open University Press
Celtic Court
22 Ballmoor
Buckingham
MK18 1XW

email: enquiries@openup.co.uk
world wide web: www.openup.co.uk

and

325 Chestnut Street
Philadelphia, PA 19106, USA

First Published 2000

A catalogue record of this book is available from the British Library

ISBN   0 335 20026 5 (pb)   0 335 20027 3 (hb)

Library of Congress Cataloging-in-Publication Data
Wilton, Tamsin.
  Sexualities in health and social care: a textbook / Tamsin Wilton with
  cartoons by the author.
    p. cm.
  Includes bibliographical references and index.
  ISBN 0-335-20026-5 (pb) – ISBN 0-335-20027-3 (hb)
  1. Social work with gays. 2. Gays–Medical care. 3. Sexual orientation.
4. Homophobia. I. Title.
HV1449.W55 2000
362.8–dc21   99–056511

Typeset by Graphicraft Limited, Hong Kong
Printed in Great Britain by Biddles Ltd, Guildford and King's Lynn

For my father, who has a Cornishman's distrust of gender roles and – like the elephant's child – an insatiable curiosity. I am grateful that he taught me both, although I am sure he sometimes regrets doing so!

contents

8 Sexuality and the family   109

9 Sexuality and public policy   131

acknowledgements

Any faults and omissions in this book are, of course, my own responsibility. However, although the physical act of writing required a mere two years, the process of research took much longer. Whether facilitating safe sex groups, lecturing to my students, collecting conference papers and articles about lesbian and gay health, videoing yet another television documentary on the gay rights movement or, on one magical occasion, running a health workshop with young lesbians in a South African township, it seems as if much of my life over the past decade has been leading up to this textbook!

Of course I have amassed more intellectual and professional debts than I am able to acknowledge here. The least I can do is to thank those who made a direct contribution to the process of writing; whether in terms of sharing their research with me, offering technical support, drawing my attention to obscure articles or casting a critical specialist eye over particular chapters. They include Rita Das, Gill Dunne, Mary Stewart, Carly Hall, Jennie Naidoo, Judy Orme, Len Doyal, Lesley Doyal, Helen de Pinho, the workers at the Triangle Project, Capetown (especially Nicci Stein and Funeka Soldaat), Gill Barrett, Gudrun Limbrick, Hazel Platzer, Dave Watkins, Hilary Lindsay, Liz Lloyd, Jeanelle de Gruchy, Lisa Saffron, Grindl Dockery, Rosie Ilett, Patricia Stevens, Simon Wright, Lyn Jennings, Adrian Booth, Nancy Worcester, Gisela Dutting, Jayne Mugglestone, Karen Hardman, Tara Kaufmann, Celia Kitzinger, Clare Farquhar, Maeve Landman, Gaynor Harper, Tati Howell and Karin Lindeqvist of the Medusa Kvinnobokhandeln in Stockholm.

For regularly picking me up, dusting me off and helping me to get back in the saddle, thanks to Stephanie Keeble, Norma Daykin, Lorraine Ayensu, Hilary Lindsay, Judy Orme, Kim Hastings, Lesley Doyal and my son and good friend, Tom Coveney. Thanks to the Bristol Women and Health Research Group and the Women's Writing Group for the yummy suppers and to members of the British Sociological Association Lesbian Studies Group for that rare thing, supportive and informed criticism. Thanks to LesBeWell (now sadly defunct), the Terrence Higgins Trust, AVERT, the Lesbian Information Service and the lesbian steering group for Sheffield Health for providing much valuable information, and to Molly Gilchrist for rescuing me from a variety of IT crises. Thanks to Andrea, Stephanie and Chrissie for allowing me to poach their computers without warning at moments of emergency, and to Rowan Gwedhen for helping me to take my first steps into the web. At Open University Press, Joan Malherbe's unfailing efficiency and courtesy provided a much appreciated antidote to authorial trauma.

A long overdue thank you to the brave crowd at Gay's The Word who somehow manage to keep us all supplied with books despite the best efforts of Her Majesty's Customs. Without their dedication to the practicalities of free speech, books like this one would be even more difficult to write. I must also say a particularly warm thank you to my lesbian and gay students, so dedicated to their own work in health and social care, who keep reminding me that this matters.

Finally, the greatest debt is to Jacinta Evans of Open University Press, who kept faith during her own transition to motherhood, and through what turned out to be an unexpectedly bumpy ride, and to Lesley Doyal, without whose rigorous and unfailingly sensitive editorial eye the whole thing might have ended up in the dustbin. Words are not enough.

how to use this book

This book is primarily intended to be useful to students in the health and social care professions; social workers, nurses, midwives, physiotherapists, radiographers, youth workers and those working in occupational health, health visiting, community nursing, mental health, residential care and other sectors of this vast and important professional arena. It also contains much of interest to medical students, as well as to students of less applied subjects such as social policy, sociology or psychology. It is designed to be appropriate for use in both basic and post-basic training, and to be helpful whether used as a classroom text or by the individual reader.

As we shall see, lack of information and understanding about human sexual diversity is widespread in health and social care, and this has potentially serious consequences for the well-being of lesbian, gay or bisexual service users and practitioners. Study after study has found that this topic is seriously neglected in basic and post-basic training, thereby undermining the ability of staff to respond effectively to the growing demand for change.

This textbook is the first of its kind. Because of this, it departs somewhat from the usual textbook formula. Much of the material here is new, and makes innovative links between research findings and practice implications. You will also find that it strays into some unfamiliar areas – the humanities, cultural studies or lesbian and gay studies, for example – simply because much that is taken for granted within these disciplines has not yet percolated through to professional education.

What this book is about

The primary aim is to support improvements in service delivery to lesbians, gay men and bisexuals by offering a foundation of sound information to be laid down during training. Crucially, as well as offering information about lesbian, gay and bisexual lives, it takes a more critical perspective on sexuality generally. In other words, rather than assuming heterosexuality as the norm, *all* sexualities are seen as being in need of explanation. This approach, although fairly time-worn in many disciplines, is a new one in the health and social care literature. It offers uniquely important insights into questions of health and well-being, since it enables us to pin-point the significance of heterosexuality (as well as homosexuality), something which is obscured by treating it as the norm.

The approach throughout is based on a model of professionalism and ethical practice that is concerned with human rights and human need, and this is underpinned by the recognition that what is good for lesbian, gay or bisexual service users is good for all.

What this book is not about

This book does not follow the model of 'sexuality' commonly used in nursing handbooks. It will not tell you how to counsel patients eager to resume sexual activity after heart surgery, nor how to reduce the rate of teenage pregnancies. It may, however, enable you to carry out such tasks in a more sensitive and appropriate manner. There is little here about the biology of human sexuality, about reproductive technologies or the clinical manifestations of various disorders of sexual function. In this book, 'sexuality' refers to sexual identity or orientation, and its consequences for health and social care practice, although sexual behaviours are also discussed.

The exercises

Each chapter is followed by a relevant exercise. These are intended to reinforce what you have learned by offering an opportunity to strengthen your understanding by making use of new knowledge. However, some of them are also designed to help you reach a clearer understanding of yourself, your own attitudes and beliefs, and the extent to which these may impact on your ability to do your job effectively. This is because sexuality is a very emotive topic, and one where personal feeling and prejudice is at least as important as rational thinking. As Carol Vance puts it, 'When we come to sex, our minds grind to a halt: normal distinctions become incomprehensible, and ordinary logic flies out the window' (Vance 1988: 17). If an exercise can help you to recognise the point at which your ordinary logic 'flies out the window', you then have the opportunity to reflect on the consequences of this and to develop strategies for dealing with it, in line with the requirements of reflexive practice.

The exercises can all be successfully carried out by the lone reader, but their outcomes may be enriched if they are done with small groups of people – about five or six for preference. None of them requires any equipment beyond scrap paper and something to write with, and they do not have 'right' or 'wrong' answers.

The sexual orientation of the reader

As a lesbian myself, I know how irritating it is when books like this one assume that all their readers will be heterosexual. However, not all heterosexuals are ignorant about lesbian and gay issues, any more than all lesbians, gay men and bisexuals are necessarily well-informed. Whatever your sexuality, I hope that you will find much here that is new to you. Some of the exercises will have a very different impact depending on the sexuality of the person engaged in them, and where I believe this to be the case I have suggested alternative approaches. It can be fun, as well as informative, to try both approaches! A word of caution. If a colleague 'comes out' to you whilst doing these exercises, do not assume that you have the right to 'out' them to anyone else. This is privileged information that still has the potential to harm, and you must check with your colleague how far they want that information to go.

A note on terminology

One reason why it is so difficult to write about sexuality is that the available language is always inadequate and often offensive. In order to write this book at all I have had to make choices about which words to use, and these need to be explained.

The word 'homosexual' is one that many gay people dislike. With its origins in nineteenth-century sexology, it carries strong overtones of pathology and medicalisation. I have therefore generally avoided using it except in those circumstances where the alternatives are too clumsy. On the other hand, despite grumbles from those who think a lovely word was 'spoilt' when homosexuals adopted it, the word *gay* has been in the lexicon of sexual slang since the seventeenth century (Grahn 1984; Stewart 1995). *Lesbian* derives from 'Lesbos', the Greek island where Sappho lived. One of the most important writers of ancient Greece (Plato called her 'the tenth Muse'), Sappho wrote love poems addressed to women, giving rise to a long tradition of referring to love between women as 'Sapphic' or 'Lesbian' love (Balmer 1984; Wilton 1995).

Members of the lesbian and gay community are often highly sensitised to the significance of naming, and there are literally dozens of self-chosen labels. I use 'lesbian' and 'gay man' for preference, since these are the terms currently in wide use in and by the community itself.

Bisexuality is not often specifically mentioned in this book. This is not out of any desire to exclude bisexuals. However, the marginalisation of bisexuals within the dominant culture is determined by the 'homosexual' rather than the 'heterosexual' component of their sexualities. Moreover, the concept of bisexuality is often used by those who wish to reinforce the idea that there is something 'real' about dividing people up into homosexual or heterosexual. In this strategy, 'bisexual' becomes what is called a 'residual category', a kind of theoretical rag bag into which you simply toss anything that does not neatly fit your schema. There are, therefore, compelling theoretical reasons for not falling back on the 'lesbian, gay and bisexual' formula, so I have refered to bisexuals only where the context demands it.

Similarly, although some transgendered people have successfully argued a case for inclusion in lesbian, gay and bisexual communities (Califia 1997), an identity constructed around deeply felt unhappiness with one's biological sex is different in kind from one constructed around same-sex desire. There is not enough space here to pay adequate attention to the complex and rapidly changing issues of transsexualism and transgender. Readers who wish to find out more about these questions are referred to the growing body of literature (see, for example, Ekins and King 1996; Califia 1997; Ekins 1997; Griggs 1998; Halberstam and Volcano 1999).

As will become clear in the discussions that follow, sexual identity is not a fixed or static concept. People may change sexual identity, the same behaviour may have different significance at different historical times or in different cultures, and the boundaries between 'gay' and 'straight' are in any case blurred and unstable. It is really only possible to use 'gay', 'lesbian' or 'bisexual' to refer to people who have adopted those names for themselves, and that is how such terms are used here. Also used regularly is one gay subcultural term that has moved into the mainstream, 'coming out'. This, together with its opposite, 'closeted', which refers to someone who has not 'come out of the closet', is now widely understood to mean acknowledging one's sexual orientation openly. Of course, this is not a once-in-a-lifetime event; lesbian, gay and bisexual people must choose where, when and to whom they entrust this information on a daily basis (Farquhar 1999).

Although names and concepts may shift, discrimination against individuals whose erotic interactions are with members of their own sex is real, and has 'real life' consequences. Laying claim to a sexual identity is also profoundly significant to individuals and to groups. It is important in any discussion of sexuality to hold on to both perceptions; that the hetero/homo divide is a social, political and cultural artefact *and yet* has real power to shape the lives of millions. This is somewhat similar to other notions, such as class, for example; we no longer believe that working-class people are biologically inferior to middle-class people, yet we recognise that massive differences in lifestyle and life chances result from the class system (Giddens 1997).

The literature

It is because 'homosexuality' has been the subject of such powerful sanctions, and because it still tends to be contaminating by association (Plummer 1981), that the task of writing a book such as this demands rather special skills of the author. A glance at the bibliography reveals that it is not only multidisciplinary, but that it includes many sources which are not formal academic texts. This is because the formal literature 'on homosexuality' was, until recently, based on the very ideas that sociologists of sexuality now criticise. In order to understand the social construction of sexualities, you need to study the dialogue of inclusion and exclusion between the sexual mainstream and those it marginalises. My source materials therefore encompass everything from learned scientific papers on genetics to VD posters aimed at the British army, from sociology textbooks to gay magazines. Each chapter has a Further Reading section. If you want to find out more about a particular topic than I could squeeze between these covers (and I hope you will), these sections should help.

1 an introduction to sexuality, health and social care

The challenge of change

Social and cultural attitudes towards sexuality underwent a dramatic process of liberalisation during the course of the twentieth century, at least in the industrialised West. Lesbian, gay or bisexual people have benefited greatly from this process, and no longer experience the extremes of social exclusion that were the norm until a few decades ago. However, social change is seldom straightforward, indeed it generally involves extended periods of uncertainty and inconsistency. This is most certainly the case for sexuality, with tolerance existing side by side with the extremes of prejudice.

Such inconsistencies are demonstrated in the July 1999 edition of the newsletter published by Stonewall, a British group that campaigns for lesbian and gay equality. Alongside a paragraph reporting the award of an OBE to its director, Angela Mason, 'for services to homosexual rights', is an article describing events following the explosion of a nail-bomb outside a gay bar in London. The public response to the bomb speaks for itself:

> As the debris was being cleared and the families and friends began to weep and the wave of shock turned to despair and loss, the calls started to come in [to Stonewall]. 'We're so very sorry.' 'Is there anything we can do?' Tears on the switchboard . . . But then 'I've got a box of nails here, shall I send it to you?' 'They should have bombed every pub in the street.' 'Fuck off nancies.' 'Gas the queers.' They go on and on. Twenty five calls by lunchtime. These words are the second cousin of the bomb.
>
> (Fanshaw 1999: 2)

This is what confronts lesbian and gay people in the UK today; a deeply contradictory world where the Queen honours those who work for 'homosexual rights' whilst others speak and act with the most savage hatred. It does not take much imagination to recognise the damage that this unpredictable situation may cause to individual health and well-being, and this is why an informed understanding of such issues is an increasingly necessary element of good practice in health and social care.

Sexuality has long been a particularly challenging issue for health and social care workers. This is, at least in part, because it has for so long been a neglected topic in education and training. As a result, concerned individuals have been left to their own devices in dealing with the range of situations where sexuality can suddenly become pertinent. This neglect has resulted in great variations in understanding, skill and competence, as research is starting to demonstrate (Cossis Brown 1992; Stevens 1993; Farquhar 1999; Mugglestone 1999). To this must be added the fact that practitioners, just as much as their clients, must cope with the often conflicting messages that accompany social transformation.

Sexuality and professional practice

Why do health and social care professionals need to know anything about the sexuality of those for whom they care? Practitioners tend to ask this question either because they are uneasy about sexuality themselves, or because they wish to protect the privacy of those they care for, or because they believe that if they treat everyone the same, regardless of gender, age, ethnicity or sexual orientation, then there will be no problem. Looking at each of these reasons in turn, it soon becomes clear that things are not that simple.

Personal unease

Working with vulnerable people requires professionalism. This involves, among other things, dealing with inappropriate personal feelings in such a way that the care of individual patients, clients or service users is not compromised. For example, it is a normal reaction to feel fear or disgust at the sight of a living person's internal organs, and fears of this kind are perfectly reasonable. Yet it is accepted that those who deal with such injuries have a professional duty to overcome their anxiety or squeamishness effectively enough to carry out their work well.

Other kinds of fearful or disgusted reactions may be less rational; for example, negative feelings about fat people, people who are disabled or disfigured, or the very elderly. However strong such feelings may be, professionalism demands that health and social care practitioners respect the human rights of service users and endeavour to meet their needs for care to the highest possible standard. Personal anxiety, unease or disgust about some aspects of human sexuality are not acceptable reasons to remain ill-informed about something which may have implications for professional practice. We would expect someone who routinely faints at the sight of blood to choose a career other than midwifery; it is equally reasonable to expect that anyone unwilling to provide respectful care to lesbian, gay or bisexual service users should not work in health and social care. However, providing care to a high standard requires a sound knowledge-base.

Protecting privacy

In the often invasive context of health and social care environments, it is important to protect the privacy of patients and clients as much as possible. However, respect for privacy is not the same as ignoring people's needs, and if service users need support in dealing with issues of sexuality there is a clear professional responsibility to respond.

For example, a gay man recovering from major surgery may be very anxious about the implications for his sex life, but may be too embarrassed to ask directly for detailed advice. Who is the better nurse in this kind of situation, the one who tactfully offers the opportunity to discuss sex and is well-informed enough to give good advice, or the one whose concern for the patient's privacy prevents any discussion about sexual matters at all? Respect for privacy is *not* a good reason for the health or social care professional failing to develop a sound knowledge base about the range of human sexualities and the skills to put this into practice with sensitivity.

Equal care

Finally, there is the argument that treating everyone in the same way guarantees equality. Here it is important to recognise the difference between *treating everyone the same*, by offering the same high standard of care to everyone, and *treating everyone as if they were the same*, which is very different. It should go without saying that everyone is entitled to the same standard of care. However, it is impossible to give good quality care by treating everyone as if they were the same. For example, it is increasingly recognised that members of different ethnic groups have different needs, and that treating them all as if they were the same (which generally means treating everyone as if they were a member of the majority ethnic group), results in a poor standard of care.

We may be more accustomed to thinking about the importance of issues such as ethnicity in this context than we are to considering sexuality. Yet sexuality is a very significant part of our lives, our closest relationships, and our sense of who we are. People receiving professional care may well be in physical or emotional pain and are likely to feel isolated, disorientated, insecure or depressed. Such feelings are stressful enough without the added pressure of having to keep a key part of your identity and your life hidden, or having the disconcerting experience of being treated as if you were someone else. Most heterosexuals would probably feel confused, disorientated or offended, if eveyone around them behaved as if they were gay. Yet most lesbians and gay men constantly have to deal with the assumption that they are heterosexual, and have the added stress of knowing that their loving relationships may not be respected by those who are caring for them. It is just as important to acknowledge differences of sexual orientation as it is to acknowledge differences of culture. It is also important to understand that homophobia is likely to impact on the well-being of lesbian or gay service users, just as racism affects the well-being of other groups.

Starting to think about homophobia

It is a fairly common error to assume that the 'homo' in words such as 'homosexual' and 'homophobic' comes from the Latin word for man, as in '*Homo sapiens*'. In fact, it comes from the Greek root meaning 'the same', as in 'homogenous'. Similarly 'heterosexual' includes the Greek root for 'different', as in 'heterogenous'. So 'homosexual' means a sexuality of sameness, and 'homophobia' (which literally means 'fear of the same') is used to mean an irrational fear or disgust towards lesbians and/or gay men.

Research evidence demonstrates that homophobia is common among those involved in health and social care, just as it is in the wider society (see, for example, Marshall 1983; Hepburn and Gutierrez 1988; Pharr 1988; Shernoff and Scott 1988; Gomez and Smith 1990; Stern 1993; Wilton 1997a, 1997b). Although such evidence is useful, it often lacks any sense of the emotional impact that homophobic incidents may have. I would like to share an anecdote from personal experience, which illustrates some of the most characteristic elements of homophobia and its potential impact in one area of practice.

After I had presented a paper on the care of lesbian mothers at a midwifery study day, an experienced community midwife came up to me, greatly agitated, and asked what should be done with the boy babies. She explained that, since all lesbians were 'truly homophobic', they would want to 'get rid' of any boy babies they gave birth to. By 'truly homophobic' she meant 'truly man-hating'.

Her convictions remained unshaken by rational argument, and she returned to practice still believing in the infanticidal tendencies of man-hating lesbians. There is nowadays no shortage of research evidence to show that lesbian mothers are remarkably similar to non-lesbian mothers, that they love and care for their children whatever sex they might be, and that the greatest problem faced by their children is not the sexuality of their mum but the homophobia of the wider society (Alpert 1988; Rafkin 1990; Kenney and Tash 1993; Saffron 1994; Gartrell *et al.* 1996; Griffin and Mulholland 1997; Dunne 1998; Wilton 1999b). In this age of evidence-based practice, this particular midwife gave *more* credence to the homophobic myths circulating in popular culture than she did to four decades of research findings within the scientific community.

This incident, whilst extreme, flags up some of the important characteristics of homophobia. In common with other prejudices, such as anti-Semitism or racism, it is irrational. However, scholars who have studied prejudice note that homophobia is not only not *felt* to be irrational – nor are racism or anti-Semitism – but is actually felt to be *morally praiseworthy* and socially sanctioned (Pharr 1988; Comstock 1991). In order to understand homophobia then, we need to think of it not simply in psychological terms, as an expression of personal fear or disturbance, but in social, cultural and political terms as well.

It is important to recognise the socio-cultural sources of homophobic sterotypes – whether pub humour or newspaper editorials – and to take seriously the consequences of political debates around such issues as equalising the age of consent or permitting lesbians and gay men to serve in the armed forces. It is not difficult to see how many factors, from Acts of Parliament to the banter of canteen culture, may contribute to the 'sense of virtue' that one researcher found amongst violently homophobic individuals (Comstock 1991).

Another key issue reflected by this incident is that homophobia is generally not taken seriously as a professional issue. If, for example, staff express extreme racist beliefs, formal structures and procedures exist to ensure that the matter could be dealt with. Equal opportunities policies, disciplinary procedures, legislation and a national race-relations policy might all be drawn on to protect the interests of vulnerable clients. Clearly such strategies have not succeeded in eradicating racism from British society or professional practice. However, the existence of formal sanctions means that racism is at least acknowledged as the social evil that it is. Because there is, as yet, *no* formal means to protect those who are lesbian or gay from discrimination, there is no equivalent acknowledgement of the wrongness of homophobia.

The continuing invisibility of homophobia as a serious professional issue may itself have indirect consequences for well-being, as one lesbian interviewed recently in Bolton indicates: 'I feel very isolated, very isolated, yeah I do. Even I end up dismissing my own needs because I'm in an environment that dismisses my needs' (Mugglestone 1999: 67).

Such statements suggest that a wider acknowledgement of the needs of lesbian and gay service users may in itself have positive benefits in terms of general confidence, self-esteem and well-being for many individuals, whether or not they come directly to the attention of service providers.

The extreme level of misinformation demonstrated by my troubled community midwife is rare. Studies have shown that many lesbian mothers receive excellent and sensitive midwifery care, although this is not yet the norm (Stevens 1993; Stewart 1997). Nor should it be assumed that lesbian or gay service users inevitably have bad experiences. Only a few weeks after my conversation with the community midwife, a friend of mine spent many weeks in hospital with serious injuries. She was visited on a regular basis by her female partner and an assortment of cheerfully 'out' lesbians. The nurses were friendly and respectful, the other patients were openly intrigued without being offensive, and her partner was treated as next of kin with no fuss at all. The entire episode was a model of good practice from start to finish and offered encouraging evidence of a positive shift in attitude.

This brings us back to the point that opened this chapter: the contradictory nature of change. There are no hard and fast rules about homophobia. One of the hardest things for lesbians and gay men to live with is its unpredictability. There is no way of knowing when you get up in the morning whether today will be one of those days when everyone you meet returns your smile, or whether you and your partner will be spat at in the street. This element of contradiction and conflict is found at every level, from the individual to the political.

When, in the summer of 1998, a bill to equalise the age of consent for gay men finally passed its first reading in the House of Commons, this sign of general acceptance was contradicted by the hostile response of many peers. Baroness Young, for example, said on ITN that night: 'I think it signals a paedophiles' charter. I think all 16-year-old boys will be at risk'. The House of Lords promptly returned the bill to the Commons, with the age of consent amendment defeated.

When those in power do not yet know the difference between a gay man and a paedophile, when sexuality is not adequately addressed in basic training, and when it is still not safe for most lesbians and gay men to be out at work, it is not surprising that many HSC practitioners – even some of those who are themselves lesbian or gay – are ill-equipped to deal with the issue of sexuality. Faced with the quite reasonable demands of lesbian and gay service users for better and more sensitive treatment, it is now a matter of some urgency to remedy the neglect of sexuality as an issue in training.

Beginning to understand sexual diversity

There is one very significant difference between sexual orientation and characteristics such as ethnicity or age. It is usually possible to tell the difference between the very young and the very old, and attributes such as skin colour, accent or dress offer clues to culture and ethnicity. Sexual orientation is not an easily perceptible set of characteristics, and it is generally only possible to know an individual's sexuality if they want you to know. This is just as true of heterosexual women and men as it is of lesbians and gay men, although heterosexuals seldom have to think about whether or not to let people know that they are heterosexual.

This characteristic, often referred to in the literature as 'invisibility', is partly because sexual orientation is not a physical characteristic like age or skin colour, but it is also reinforced by the very real need for concealment caused by heterosexism (see below) and homophobia. Not being able to read clear signals is one simple reason why many heterosexual women and men believe that they have never come into contact with a lesbian or gay man, and this may have implications for quality of care. For example, it is not uncommon for clinicians to claim that they have never treated lesbian or gay patients, even when this assertion is statistically highly unlikely (Robertson 1993). Of course, if you genuinely believe that you have no lesbian or gay service users, you are unlikely to perceive the issue as serious or relevant to your own practice, and this in turn contributes to a wider perception of sexual orientation as a marginal issue.

Heterosexism

It may be easy to understand why it might be offensive to treat heterosexuals as if they were gay, but less easy to recognise why it might be equally offensive to treat lesbians and gay men as if they were heterosexual. This in itself is a sign that heterosexuality is, often unthinkingly, valued more highly than homosexuality. To regard heterosexuality as being better, more normal, more natural or more morally right than homosexuality is called *heterosexism*. Although different from homophobia, heterosexism also has an important impact on the delivery of health and social care. It tends to result in errors of omission – for example, designing admissions forms that assume heterosexuality by using terminology such as 'marital status' – rather than direct or indirect hostility.

Attitudes have improved in many Western societies in recent years, and it may appear that the lesbian and gay members of these societies are now fully accepted. However, although these changes have made a very real difference to the lives of many millions of people, they are still relatively superficial. For example, gay soap operas on television probably bear the same relation to general homophobia as the *Cosby Show* does to general racism.

The professional context

Researchers have found substantial evidence that lesbian and gay users of the health and social care services commonly meet with ignorance, hostility, rude and offensive behaviour and even aggression if they are open about their sexual orientation (Shernoff and Scott 1988; Stevens 1993; Dockery 1996; Sheffield Health 1996). Even where heterosexual staff are well-meaning they may be ill-informed, and this often means that service users are left with the responsibility of educating them about relevant issues or are obliged to put up with voyeuristic and intrusive questioning (Stevens 1993; Wilton 1997b).

This is a catch-22 situation. Although staff clearly need information, it is hardly surprising that their *lack* of information causes many lesbians and gay men to conceal their sexuality. Well-meaning individuals may find this frustrating, failing to understand that such concealment is often necessary for personal safety. Lesbians and gay men must constantly decide whether or not it is safe to 'come out', what the likely consequences will be, and whether or not they can trust the judgement of the other people involved. It is a question not only of predicting the responses of the person you are about to tell, but also of whether or not they are likely to tell others, and what the reaction of those unknown people may be. In the context of a hospital, a care team, a general practice, or a local authority social services unit, it can become very difficult for individuals to retain control over who knows and who does not. Since homophobia is so widespread, this lack of control can be very stressful, and has been identified as the reason why many continue to conceal their sexuality even from their general practitioners (GPs) (Somerset Health Authority 1998; Mugglestone 1999; Wilton 1999b).

Both openness and concealment carry risks for the individual concerned. If they choose to come out, they risk having to deal with negative reactions. If they choose not to, they will have to deal with the emotional costs of secrecy, and with being treated as if they are something that they are not. Both scenarios carry personal costs in terms of stress, anxiety, fear and insecurity. In the context of illness, injury or personal crisis, such an additional burden is likely to have a negative impact on an individual's ability to heal, to recover or to surmount crisis and regain strength and stability.

Religious beliefs and moral dilemmas

One important distinction between homophobia and other forms of dis-crimination is that many people believe that love between individuals of the same biological sex is *morally* wrong. It is not generally thought, even by the most disturbed racist, that to be black is an immoral act – although many racists do claim that black people are more likely to behave in an immoral way than non-black people. In contrast, many insist that simply to be gay, lesbian or bisexual is to *be* immoral.

Moreover, many believe that their religion condemns homosexuality. This moral/religious aspect of the issue may cause painful conflicts for the HSC professional who genuinely wants to offer the very best standard of care to all users of their service, but who feels that their religious or moral beliefs prohibit them from offering good care to lesbian, gay or bisexual people. There is no easy way out of this dilemma. It is an absolute requirement of professionalism that personal beliefs be set aside when they conflict with professional duty. The *sole* exception to this rule is that nurses are permitted to refuse to assist at the termination of pregnancies on religious grounds. This acceptance of duty may demand a thoughtful and open-minded re-evaluation of one's religious or moral standpoint, and it may help to seek advice from one of the lesbian and gay religious groups (for a useful directory of such groups, see Green *et al.* 1996).

Religion

Researchers have repeatedly found a clear association between homphobic attitudes and strong religious belief (Pharr 1988; Comstock 1991; Haldeman 1991; Sears 1991; Griffin *et al.* 1998), and this is as true of clinicians and health and social care professionals as it is of any other group (Stevens 1993). Sometimes, homophobic individuals opportunistically make use of what they assume to be religious doctrine in order to justify their own prejudices (Haldeman 1991). In other cases however, individuals with deeply held religious beliefs quite genuinely believe that homosexuality is forbidden by their religion.

There is a more substantial discussion of religious attitudes in later chapters. Here, it is useful to recognise that the holy writings of the world's great religions – Judaism, Christianity, Sikhism, Hinduism, Islam and Buddhism – barely mention homosexuality. The Gospels, for example, contain not a single reference to it. This is not surprising since, as one theologian points out, 'The terms *homosexual* and *heterosexual* were not developed in any language until the 1890s . . . Therefore the use of the word *homosexuality* by certain English Bible translators is an example of the extreme bias that endangers the human and civil rights of homosexual persons' (Mollenkott, cited in Pharr 1988: 3, emphasis in original). Many contemporary scholars agree that the Bible has nothing to say about homosexuality *per se*. Indeed, Helminiak concludes (1994: 108), 'the Bible takes no direct stand on the morality of . . . gay and lesbian relationships'. Where homosexual acts are mentioned, it is usually something other than the gender of the participants which is the issue (Helminiak 1994).

The same is true for other religious traditions; it is the legislative apparatus created by the administrative infrastructure of the world's religions that forbids same-sex relationships. In other words, human authority, not divine law, appears to be the issue. This interpretation remains contentious, but it is clear that religious condemnation of homosexuality is by no means as unequivocal as many assume, and that theologians have found at least as much *acceptance* of same-sex love in the world's great religious texts as rejection.

It is, therefore, no easy solution to call on religion to justify a personal belief in the immorality or unnaturalness of homosexuality. Concluding an exhaustive study into the morality of homosexuality, philosopher

Michael Ruse writes that: 'the argument that homosexuality is biologically unnatural and hence immoral, fails', and recommends that 'one ought to persuade people not to confuse their disgust . . . with moral indignation' (Ruse 1988: 196 and 291).

Implications for practice

The homophobia and heterosexism that researchers have identified within health and social care are morally and professionally indefensible. This does not mean that it is easy to shed homophobic prejudices, but it does mean that there is a clear moral as well as professional obligation to recognise them for what they are. As one psychologist recommends to clergymen, 'Even if you are unable to see the beauty and dignity of Gay people, even if you continue to believe that Gay is sinful and immoral, be good enough to tell the trusting Gay person who consults you that it is your opinion and your interpretation of your religion' (Clark 1987: 224).

For many working in the field of health and social care, religious belief offers both a source of comfort in an often stressful career and a primary motivation to care for others in this way. In other words, faith often supports the professional ethos. However, in cases where it comes into conflict with a practitioner's ability to deliver respectful and appropriate care, there is a clear obligation to prioritise professional standards over personal belief or morality. Such professional skills are best supported by developing an informed understanding of the social and cultural roots of homophobia, and by exploring *both* sides of the relevant religious debates.

---

exercise

Working alone or with a partner, write down the names of as many well-known gay men as you can think of. Give yourself ten minutes. Now do the same for well-known lesbians.

Points to think about:

- Which list is longer, and which was easier to collect? What does this tell you?

- What did it feel like writing down the names? Were you unwilling to write down any names of people you were not absolutely sure about? What does this tell you?

- If you yourself are lesbian or gay, how did it make you feel doing this exercise? Do you feel that your 'insider knowledge' is a useful professional resource, or that it may expose you to homophobia from your colleagues?

Further reading

Clark, D. (1987) *The New Loving Someone Gay*. Berkeley, CA: Celestial Arts.

Gonsiorek, J. and Weinrich, J. (eds) (1991) *Homosexuality: Research Implications for Public Policy*. London: Sage.

Green, T., Harrison, B. and Innes, J. (1996) *Not for Turning: An Enquiry into the Ex-Gay Movement*. Leeds: published by the authors.

Hawkes, G. (1996) *A Sociology of Sex and Sexuality*. Buckingham: Open University Press.

Pharr, S. (1988) *Homophobia: A Weapon of Sexism*. Little Rock: Chardon Press.

Rosenblum, R. (ed.) (1996) *Unspoken Rules: Sexual Orientation and Women's Human Rights*. London: Cassell.

Ruse, M. (1988) *Homosexuality: A Philosophical Inquiry*. Oxford: Basil Blackwell.

Weeks, J. (1985) *Sexuality and Its Discontents: Meanings, Myths and Modern Sexualities*. London: Routledge & Kegan Paul.

2 sexual orientation and its consequences

Introduction

This chapter introduces key concepts concerning sexuality and some of the most important social issues associated with **sex**, **gender** and **sexual identity**. It discusses the relationships between those aspects of sex which are biological and those which are social or cultural, and outlines the social and political situation of sexual minorities around the world.

Biological sex and social gender

One of the first questions to be asked when a baby is born is, 'Is it a boy or a girl?' Being male or female is extremely significant in all human societies, although the differences in behaviour expected of the two sexes vary widely between cultures. Ideas about what makes a 'real man' or a 'real woman' may vary quite dramatically from country to country, or from one cultural group to another within countries. In an ethnically diverse country such as Britain, there are likely to be conflicting ideas about proper female or male behaviour among different communities. Such ideas may concern dress, courtship and marriage customs, relationships between parents and children or husbands and wives, what kinds of work are appropriate for men or women, access to education and training and many other aspects of daily life. Expectations of appropriate behaviour are often so strongly *gendered* that women and men may inhabit almost completely separate spheres (Abercrombie *et al.* 1994).

So, although almost all cultures treat their male and female members as if they were very different kinds of people, different cultures stress different aspects of behaviour or appearance. Sometimes religion plays a part in this; the Sikh religion, for example, insists that adult males must refrain from cutting their hair, whilst long hair is regarded as definitively feminine in the secular West. Such rules are not always religious. For example, Europeans of all faiths have a far more relaxed attitude to men exposing their upper bodies than to women doing so, and this remains the case even in the most secular societies.

In addition to such differences between cultures, social values tend to change over time. We recognise that young adults may have quite different values to those of their grandparents or even their own parents, and this is particularly true when it comes to what is expected of the sexes. Any university or hospital canteen today, for example, is likely to be full of women wearing clothing that would have got them arrested in their great-grandparents' day.

Ideas concerning the different behaviours expected of women and men may have very little to do with biological sex. There is no biological reason why men should not wear dresses to work or why women should not enter a synagogue bare-headed. Nor, as cross-cultural studies make quite clear, is there any biological reason why men should not make excellent nurses or secretaries and women should not succeed as nuclear physicists or coal miners. The reasoning behind these different expectations is social and cultural, and it is this 'package' of social and cultural assumptions about the differences between the sexes that we call *gender*.

Anthropologists and sociologists recognise that the rules governing gender are socially, culturally and historically *contingent*; that is, that they vary from time to time and from place to place. Nevertheless, they are such a key part of the way in which most societies are organised – for example, both paid and unpaid work may be broadly divided into 'men's work' and 'women's work' – that there is a tendency to assume that familiar gender rules are natural, right and proper.

Depending on whether the society in question is religious or secular, these rules may be explained as the will of God or a law of nature. For example, the Christian Church held for many centuries that the social rules governing the behaviour of women and men were ordained by God, as is clear from this thirteenth-century passage written by St Thomas Aquinas:

> Male and female are joined together in humans, not only on account of the necessity for generation . . . but also for domestic life, in which there are different jobs for the man and the woman, and in which the man is the head of the woman.
>
> (Cited in Cadden 1993: 193)

As the power of the Church waned in Europe, and as belief in science replaced belief in religious explanations of the universe, the same social rules were now reinterpreted as laws of 'nature'. For example, this is how the Victorian writer Walter Bagehot responded to the campaign to give women the vote:

> the attempt to alter the present relation of the sexes is . . . not an attempt to break the yoke of mere convention; it is a struggle against Nature; a war undertaken to reverse the very conditions against which not man alone, but all mammalian species have reached their present development.
>
> (Cited in Martin 1987: 32)

The words of Aquinas and Bagehot help to explain why men who behave in ways that are traditionally reserved for women, or vice versa, have historically been condemned as either ungodly or unnatural.

More recently, developments in global communications and transport have brought widespread exposure to the beliefs and customs of many different cultures and societies. It is now evident that there is an almost infinite number of variations on gender roles, and that each set of rules has its own benefits and drawbacks. It is no longer possible to believe that the social rules governing gendered behaviour have their roots in biology, nor that there is one right way of organising 'male' and 'female' roles in society.

However, because gender is such a fundamental element of social organisation it tends to be equally fundamental in the process of socialisation and the development of a sense of self. In other words, it matters very much to individuals whether they themselves are female or male, and that they are able to tell whether others are female or male (Ekins 1997; Griggs 1998). Social transformations in gender roles may therefore be experienced as very disturbing, and this may lead individuals and groups to seek reassurance in the belief that these roles are determined by nature or ordained by God. So it is not uncommon, even today, to find that non-typical gender behaviour (for example, a woman who chooses not to have children or a man who gives up work to become a 'househusband') may be described as 'unnatural'.

Gender and sexual practice

At the root of the social organisation of gender lie a set of assumptions about biological sex and its relationship with sexual behaviour and repro-duction. Again, such beliefs are culturally and historically contingent. During the Middle Ages in Europe, for example, it was thought that the female genitals were exactly the same as male genitals, only in women they were underdeveloped and had not grown outside the body. The penis and scrotum were thought to be a vagina and uterus which had turned inside out and taken up position outside the body rather than inside (Sawday 1995). The male body was thought to be more perfect than the female body, because it had undergone this additional stage of development.

Great social significance is attached to sexual anatomy, but the ideas and beliefs about gender and sexuality, which are probably taken for granted by most people in Britain today, are in fact the product of history and social change, rather than the inevitable consequence of biology or anatomy. There are almost certainly some aspects of our current thinking about sex and sexuality that future generations will find just as laughable as we find the medieval idea that the uterus is an undeveloped scrotum.

It is difficult to stand outside a world view that we take for granted and to disentangle the various strands which contribute to these ideas. They include elements from biology, from Darwinian thinking on natural selection, from Judaeo-Christian religious tradition, from popular versions of Freudian psychology and from shared beliefs about what constitutes socially acceptable behaviour. These different elements, themselves com-plex, weave together to produce a picture in which gender and sexual behaviour seem to us to be very closely linked.

Bodies and desires

To be female or to be male is to have a body with specific characteristics. A female body has a vagina, uterus, ovaries and distinctive breasts. A male body has a penis, testes, scrotum and only vestigial breasts. There is assumed to be a specific reproductive and evolutionary purpose behind these characteristics. A vagina and uterus are 'meant' to be penetrated by a penis, so it is generally assumed that woman describes a person who will instinctively *want* her vagina to be penetrated by a penis, and who will experience this as sexual desire. Similarly, a man is assumed to be a person who will *want* to put his penis into a vagina, and who will experi-ence desire for this to take place.

In other words, there is a very strong assumption that human beings are *designed for* heterosexual intercourse much as an electrical plug and socket are designed to fit together. This view of sex and desire may be described as *functionalist*. Although bodies demonstrably *are* suited to their reproductive function, it is a huge leap to claim that desires and behaviour therefore also follow function. To do so requires that we ignore human characteristics such as inventiveness, emotionality and free will.

According to this functionalist view, a man is by definition someone who is sexually attracted to women, and vice versa. This is why so many people – and they include homosexuals as well as heterosexuals, scientists as well as lay people – believe that a man who is attracted to other men must be in some way woman-like or feminine, and a woman who is attracted to other women must be man-like or masculine. Thus, the Campaign for Press and Broadcasting Freedom, in a survey of press representations of lesbians and gay men over a 14-day period, found words such as 'bearded', 'burly' and 'boiler-suited' routinely used to generalise about lesbians (Armitage *et al.* 1987).

The functionalist model of sexuality that underpins such stereotypes is itself based on a misunderstanding of evolution (Gould 1995). The 'plug-and-socket' model can only be made to work by ignoring some characteristics of human biology and concentrating on others. If a female body is designed to be penetrated by a penis, why is the clitoris not *inside* the vagina? Similarly, if the male body is designed only to get sexual pleasure from penetrating a vagina, then why is the sexually sensitive prostate gland located *inside* the rectum? If we are to decide what kinds of sexual coupling are 'natural' by examining the sexual anatomy of the human body, the argument that penis-in-vagina sex is the *only* kind of sex we are designed for is not very persuasive. This, in turn, suggests that functionalist arguments for the biological naturalness of this form of heterosexual activity may themselves be strongly influenced by social and cultural factors.

Such ideas are widespread and deeply held, and it is often difficult to see them for what they are – beliefs held by a particular social group at a particular time in its history. To take another common line of thought, many people believe that heterosexuality is more 'natural' than homosexuality because *opposites attract*. Here a law has been borrowed from physics and applied to human behaviour as an explanatory metaphor. Yet it really makes very little sense to think of women and men as 'opposite'. They do not carry opposite electromagnetic charges, they are not located at opposite ends of any kind of spectrum, indeed they are not, in any meaningful sense, the opposite of each other at all, simply different in certain ways. Yet, to speak of heterosexual attraction as if it were similar to the electromagnetic attraction between positive and negative is very common.

Widespread, taken-for-granted beliefs of this kind may shape perceptions of lesbian and gay relationships as well as heterosexual ones. For example, there is a fairly common assumption that, in any relationship between two men or two women, one must take the role of the 'opposite' sex for desire to be generated. One of the couple (whatever their biological sex) is expected to play the part of 'the man' by doing a man's job, dressing in a masculine way, fixing things around the house and taking the 'dominant' role in sex, while the other is expected to play the role of 'the little woman' by cooking, cleaning, being emotional and taking the 'submissive' role in sex.

Of course, there are relationships where roles do divide neatly in this way, but there are just as many where this does not happen, and this is as true of lesbian and gay couples as it is of their heterosexual counterparts (Dunne 1997).

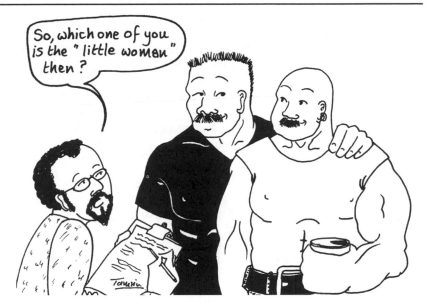

Sexual practice and sexual identity

It is because the division into two genders is such an important structural feature of society, and because there is such a strong association between experiencing heterosexual desire and being a 'proper' woman or man, that sexual preference itself has become a significant social division. So significant is it in our own historical time that the *gender* to which an individual is primarily attracted results in the social ascription of a *sexual identity* as homosexual, heterosexual or bisexual.

What is more, because the cultural link between gender role and specific aspects of sexual behaviour is so strong, there is also an assumption that *any* sexual coupling will follow a gendered division of labour. An 'active' partner does the man's job of penetrating, and a 'passive' partner plays the part of the woman and is penetrated. Since penetrating someone else is so closely linked with masculinity, it is thought to be unnatural and effeminate for a man to allow himself to be penetrated, as this is the sexual role proper to women. Indeed some cultures regard only this kind of 'passive' homosexual behaviour as shameful, believing that the 'active' partner retains his masculine status (Lancaster 1995).

In fact, it is not the case that two men will always take these complementary roles during sexual encounters or relationships. Whether they do or not seems largely to depend on the expectations of the society in which they live and on their own personal preference. Indeed, some gay men living in the West have very egalitarian sexual values and attach great importance to their ability to move beyond the restrictions of traditional active/passive roles (Watney 1987; Dyer 1989). Moreover, sexual activity between two men, like that between any couple, is not restricted to, and does not always include, penetration (Fitzpatrick *et al.* 1990).

If it is difficult to make male homosexuality fit into a heterosexual mould, lesbians have presented even greater problems. After all, two men between them have the right anatomical equipment to enable hetero-sexuals to imagine a recognisable form of intercourse taking place. The idea of sex taking place between two women, in the absence of anything resembling a penis, has long thrown heterosexual theorists into confusion. I remember giggling in the school playground at the following anonymous limerick:

An eager gay man from Khartoum
Took a lesbian up to his room
They argued all night
Over who had the right
To do what, and with which, and to whom.

The humour lay in the implication that, although there was a man and a woman in that room in Khartoum, since one of them was a *gay* man (and hence effeminate) and the other was a lesbian (and hence mas-culine), it was impossible to imagine what kind of sexual act they might perform.

Heterosexual theorists have tended to bypass their confusion about lesbian sexual behaviour in one of two ways; either by proposing that some sort of penis *must* exist, or that, since there is no penis, then what happens does not count as sex. The first proposal has led to the assertion that lesbians must use dildos, or that they have an elongated clitoris, which they use as if it were a penis (Barale 1991). This rather odd belief, which has never been supported by empirical research, was widely held by clinicians right up to the 1980s (Hemmings 1986). This is intriguing, since it suggests that the social and cultural construction of lesbians as masculine carries such weight that it may even override the rules of evidence-based scientific 'objectivity' governing clinical practice.

The second position – that nothing can be real sex unless there is a penis involved – leads to the assertion that, since they never experience 'real' sex, lesbians are immature and childish, as well as deeply frustrated and unhappy. This is the thinking that lies at the root of the common heterosexual male fantasy that a lesbian who experiences 'proper' sex with a skilled male lover will be converted to heterosexuality.

We tend to assume that fantasy may be easily distinguished from reality. Novelists deal in fantasy, academics and doctors in reality. For example, when 'lesbian' sex scenes are published in pornographic magazines, as they often are (see Wilton 1996), few believe they are witnessing the 'real thing'. However, ideas put forward by serious academics are more likely to be taken at face value. Philosopher Roger Scruton describes lesbian sex as something that never really takes place at all: 'there is an extremely poignant, often helpless, sense of being at another's mercy . . . the lesbian

can only wait, and wish, and pray to the gods with . . . troubled fervour'
(Scruton 1986: 35).

By the time these words were written, plenty of lesbians had taken
part in large-scale sexological research studies or had written openly
about their lives and relationships. This body of material was readily
available and demonstrated not only that lesbians in general appeared to
be *more* satisfied with their sexual relationships than non-lesbian women
(Hite 1976), but also that a small but increasing number of women who
had previously lived active heterosexual lives were making a conscious
choice to live as lesbians (Darty and Potter 1984; Abbott and Love 1985).
Scruton had chosen to ignore a significant body of evidence, which strongly
suggested that many women find sexual relationships with other women
perfectly satisfactory, choosing instead to present his own unsubstantiated
views as fact. As an academic with an established reputation, his words
carry considerable weight and hence may help to perpetuate negative
attitudes towards this group of women.

Changing identities?

Since the nineteenth century it has been widely assumed that individuals
are pretty much fixed in their orientation towards either male or female
partners. As we shall see, many theories have been put forward to explain
the origin or cause of sexual identity, but most of these theories have
taken for granted that there are different kinds of people – heterosexual,
homosexual or bisexual – and that these divisions are real and unchang-
ing. You are either one or other of the possible options, and your sexual
identity is as much a part of who you are as your hair colour or your
height. Yet, recent research has produced a substantial amount of evidence
to suggest that sexual identity is, in fact, not so clear-cut.

The first piece of research to challenge the notion of fixed sexual identity was a major American study published in 1948 by pioneering sex
researcher Alfred Kinsey. Kinsey interviewed over 18,000 subjects, and
the published study found that 37 per cent of his male interviewees had
experienced sexual encounters leading to orgasm with another man at
least once, although only 4 per cent described themselves as exclusively
homosexual (Kinsey *et al.* 1948). In 1970, the American sociologist Laud
Humphreys published a detailed study of men who met other men in
public toilets for casual sex. Despite the general assumption that their
behaviour indicated that these men were homosexual, Humphreys found
that the majority of his interviewees thought of themselves as heterosexual
and many were happily married (Humphreys 1970).

More recently, there have been many studies into the sexual behaviour
of men who do identify as gay (e.g. Davies *et al.* 1990, 1993; Fitzpatrick
et al. 1990). This research has shown not only that large numbers of men
have sex with other men while continuing to think of themselves as
heterosexual, but also that a substantial minority of men who identify as
gay continue to have occasional sex with women. It seems that, contrary

to general expectation, individuals do not necessarily base their own sexual identity on behaviour or desire. In other words, when someone calls themself lesbian, gay, bisexual or heterosexual, this does not necessarily depend on who they have sex with.

Researchers responded to these findings by coining the term 'men who have sex with men' in an attempt to highlight the distinction between behaviour and identity. One important British study, Project SIGMA, summed up the situation in their report to the Department of Health:

> there remains an abiding assumption . . . that homosexual men and heterosexual men form two hermetic communities . . . despite the fact that there are women and men who will affirm the identity 'bisexual', there are many more who, terming themselves gay or straight, will engage, regularly or infrequently, in sex with partners of either gender.
>
> (Davies *et al.* 1990: 143)

To complicate matters still further, recent research indicates that individuals may change their sexual identity over the course of a lifetime, and that this seems to be especially true for women (Hall Carpenter Archives 1989; Barrett 1990; National Lesbian and Gay Survey 1992; Whisman 1996; Wilton 1999b). A woman may grow up heterosexual, marry and have a family, and may then go on to adopt a lesbian identity and form her intimate relationships with women. Another may spend a large part of her life living as a lesbian, and then may form a relationship with a man and take on a heterosexual identity (Clausen 1990; Menasche 1999). Because sexual identity carries such a weight of social expectation, an individual whose identity shifts may experience massive upheaval in her life, as lesbian writer Jan Clausen found when she fell in love with a man:

> I was . . . plunged into an experience of profound discontinuity, my basic sense of who I was called into question . . . It's a shock to find myself once again facing problems I dimly recall from my heterosexual youth, built-in inequalities I thought I'd cleverly sidestepped by choosing my own kind . . . The emotional disparities are equally unsettling.
>
> (Clausen 1990: 13–14)

It is clear from these accounts that such experiences do not fit into the category of bisexuality. Indeed, bisexuality is itself a complex question, about which there is much debate and disagreement (see, for example, Ault 1996; Whisman 1996).

In conclusion, there is much that remains uncertain about the relationship between sexual behaviour, gender and sexual identity. Although the *social* division into homosexual and heterosexual carries a great deal of weight, it does not seem to be either an accurate or an adequate description of the experiences it is supposed to define.

Sexuality and stigma

One of the reasons why our knowledge about sexuality is so inadequate is that sex has traditionally been a highly sensitive area of human social life, and one surrounded with prohibitions and taboos. Until very recently, those brave enough to carry out research into human sexual behaviours, or to question the social organisation of sexuality, were regarded with great suspicion. This was true of sexuality in general, but even more so for homosexuality. Even today, research into lesbian and gay issues is fraught with difficulties; as British sociologist Ken Plummer makes clear, 'it is hard to get funding, people would like to stop us doing our work . . . people look with suspicion on gay and lesbian causes, there is employment discrimination and so on' (Plummer 1992: 12).

However, the stigma attached to homosexuality is certainly less extreme than it was in the recent past, at least in Europe. A respected scholar, writing about male homosexuality in 1928, described it in tones which now seem more suited to the pages of a horror story:

> It throbs in our huge cities . . . It once sat, clothed in Imperial purple, on the throne of the Roman Caesars, crowned with the tiara on the [papal] chair of St. Peter . . . Yet no one dares to speak of it; or if they do, they bate their breath, and preface their remarks with maledictions . . . I can hardly find a name which will not seem to soil this paper.
>
> (Symonds 1984: 5–6)

These words will seem rather extreme to a contemporary British reader, who is able to watch gay characters sympathetically portrayed in television soaps and who may even have voted for an openly gay Member of Parliament. Yet it is important to remember that these traditional attitudes continue to influence the attitudes of many in British society and that, in many other countries, homosexuality remains illegal or is subject to extreme repression.

Civil and human rights: violence

The British charity, War on Want, reports that homosexuality remains illegal in many parts of the world, including Singapore, Jamaica, Zimbabwe, Bangladesh, Malaysia, India, Pakistan, Algeria and Chile. The situation is particularly dangerous in countries under Islamic law, such as Iran (where punishment for being accused of homosexual acts include whipping, cutting off of hands or feet or stoning to death) or Pakistan (where life imprisonment and/or a beating of up to 100 lashes are the common penalty). In China, homosexuality is considered to be a foreigners' disease and there are reliable accounts of attempts to 'cure' gay men with electric shocks, while in Ecuador gay men have been killed by death squads.

Agencies working in the field have struggled to get such abuses of human rights recognised. The director of War on Want, Margaret Lynch, was 'quite shocked to discover that no other UK aid organisation funds lesbian and gay projects abroad' (War on Want 1996), whilst it took 17 years of pressure from lesbian and gay activists to persuade Amnesty International to recognise human rights abuses on grounds of sexual orientation as part of its mandate (Rosenblum 1996). Even the international movement for recognition of women's human rights has been reluctant to acknowledge lesbians, as a number of commentators are now pointing out. Charlotte Bunch (Rosenblum 1996: vii) writes:

> Every person who upholds the right of women to human dignity and bodily integrity must ask why is this issue so difficult to support? Why after so many years does such profound prejudice, ignorance and discrimination against women solely on the ground of their sexual orientation continue to flourish?

Bunch goes on to insist that, rather than being a 'special issue', lesbian and gay rights are an integral element of *all* human rights, since it makes little sense to fight for human beings to have the right to everything *except* the freedom of sexual expression. Nor is it possible to establish respect for universal human rights if you exclude any group from your definition of 'universal'. She concludes, 'If the human rights of any group are left behind, the human rights of all are incomplete' (Rosenblum 1996: viii).

Although the situation is better in Britain than in some other parts of the world, human rights observers have concluded that lesbian and gay citizens are still subject to prejudice and discriminatory treatment (Palmer 1996). Although they pay the same taxes as anyone else, they do not have equal protection under the law, nor do they have the same benefits as heterosexual citizens (Galloway 1983; Palmer 1996). There is no employment protection – it is not against the law for a homophobic employer to dismiss someone simply because they are lesbian or gay. However long term they may be, lesbian and gay partnerships do not have the rights associated with heterosexual marriage in terms of inheritance, pension entitlement, life insurance coverage or tax benefits. The end result is that the lesbian and gay section of the community financially subsidises heterosexuals to a significant extent, a situation about which some trades unions are becoming increasingly concerned.

The English and Scottish legal systems have been among the last in Europe to hold out against an equal age of consent and to continue the prohibition on lesbians and gay men serving in the armed forces – and, despite recent changes, continue to discriminate on grounds of sexual orientation. Legislation such as Section 28 of the 1988 Local Government Act (which prohibits local authorities funding the 'promotion of homosexuality'), whilst generally agreed to be unworkable in the courts (Colvin and Hawksely 1989), gives a strong public signal that homosexuality is unacceptable.

An American researcher, Gary Comstock, carried out an important study into the motives of those convicted of violent attacks on lesbians and gay men. He concluded that the most important distinction between homophobic assault and other forms of unprovoked violence (such as racist beatings) was that violence towards lesbians and gay men is considered socially acceptable among large sectors of the population. Far from feeling remorse for injuring (and in some cases murdering) another human being, Comstock found that many of the perpetrators maintained what he called a 'sense of virtue' concerning their crimes (Comstock 1991: 22). Seen in this context, legislation that appears to sanction discrimination may have consequences far beyond what was intended by those who drafted it.

Lesbians and gay men are commonly denied the basic human right to freedom from violent assault. Homophobic violence – unprovoked attacks on those believed by the perpetrators to be homosexual – is characterised by its extreme nature. It is both widespread and extraordinarily vicious. The United States Justice Department keeps statistics on 'bias crimes', that is crimes committed out of prejudice such as racism or homophobia on the part of the perpetrator. These statistics indicate that the commonest form of bias crime in the US is unprovoked violent assault against gay men (Comstock 1991). As one spokeswoman for the American lesbian and gay community wrote:

> Our claims to full humanity, to civil rights and the legal status of citizenship, have met strong and organized resistance. We are, according to even the Reagan Justice Department, the most frequent victims of hate crimes: murders, assaults, robberies, arsons, vandalism, threats and harassments.
>
> (Segrest 1995: 79)

The particularly vicious nature of this kind of assault is also evident in Britain from press accounts of murders in which gay men are the victims. This has led some psychologists to posit that the perpetrators are young men so disturbed by their own homosexual impulses that they are driven to violence (Pharr 1988; Shernoff and Scott 1988; Comstock 1991). US hospital records speak for themselves:

> Melissa Mertz, co-ordinator of the Victims of Violent Assault Assistance Program of Bellevue Hospital in Manhattan, says that 'attacks against gay men were the most heinous and brutal I encountered.' She continues, 'They frequently involved torture, cutting, mutilation, and beating, and showed the absolute intent to rub out the human being because of his sexual orientation.' . . . Other sources concur with this evidence of overkill and excessive mutilation. In a study of autopsy findings by physicians, one psychiatrist stated that 'multiple and extensive wounds are not uncommon in the fury of' anti-homosexual murder.
>
> (Comstock 1991: 46–7)

Although disturbing, homophobic murder remains rare. However, a survey of London lesbian and gay teenagers found that verbal abuse and being beaten up were experiences shared by the young men and women in the group. The majority of the mixed-sex sample (58 per cent) had been verbally abused and a substantial minority (21 per cent) had been beaten up, with the percentages being the same for young men and women (London Gay Teenage Group 1984). A more recent survey found that one in three gay men and one on four lesbians had experienced at least one violent assault in the previous five years, leading the future Home Secretary, Jack Straw to conclude that 'gay people are . . . disproportionately likely to be the victims of harassment and attack' (Mason and Palmer 1997).

Just as the fear of rape influences the behaviour of all women, so the fear of homphobic assault influences the behaviour of all lesbians and gay men. One young London lesbian told researchers, 'I have to conform to a feminine straight stereotype. If I do not I might get beaten up for being a lesbian. Just the violence. The violence is the main thing' (London Gay Teenage Group 1984: 144). Another lesbian who took part in a recent survey of lesbian, gay and bisexual lives in Bristol commented, 'As a tenant on an estate it is a matter of life and death (literally) survival to stay in the closet' (Wilton 1999a). Comstock (1991: 14) concludes, 'That one could without provocation be physically attacked on the street, at home, in one's place of social gathering [is] in lesbian and gay neighbourhoods an experience so recurrent that one live[s] with the hope of avoiding it while realizing that it could easily happen.'

Worryingly there is evidence that the police, who should offer some degree of protection against homophobic violence, may themselves ignore or even contribute to it. There are many cases on public record in Australia, Britain, the United States and mainland European countries, where police officers have carried out homophobic beatings and even murders (Connell 1987; Greenberg 1988; Comstock 1991; Mason and Palmer 1997). Courts, government bodies and the police themselves may ignore, deny or belittle homophobic violence and offenders often go unpunished (Connell 1987; Greenberg 1988; Cruikshank 1992; Gomez *et al.* 1995). Australian academic Bob Connell reports 'an entertainment for off duty policemen [in Adelaide] which consisted of bashing homosexual men and throwing them in the River Torrens' (Connell 1987: 12), a practice which resulted in the death of at least one gay man, Dr George Duncan. Connell concludes, 'Homosexual men have reason to fear assault in public places – and one of the main groups they have to fear are the police.'

The police in Britain are responding to community pressures to acknowledge this problem, and are taking steps, in consultation with local lesbian, gay and bisexual groups, to tackle homophobic violence. London's Metropolitan Police Force has taken the lead, recruiting lesbian and gay officers, appointing special liaison officers and working in cooperation with the local community and the lesbian and gay press, whilst other regions have introduced schemes to monitor assaults and provide appropriate support to victims. A survey into homophobic violence carried out by Stonewall (Mason and Palmer 1996: 84) found that, 'In the last five years, 41 out of

43 police forces have adopted new management policies which recognise the principle of equal treatment for lesbians and gay men.' However, there is still a long way to go. Moreover, some recent surveys have indicated that, while some police forces in the UK have improved the service they offer to gay men, they remain considerably less sensitive to lesbian and bisexual women (Mason and Palmer 1996; Sheffield Health 1996; Mugglestone 1999; Wilton 1999a).

Heterosexuality as social norm

We have seen that homosexuality remains stigmatised in Western societies and that lesbians and gay men may be the victims of verbal abuse or violence. Both stigma and violence are *negative sanctions*, which have the effect of reinforcing social norms. In this case, the negative sanctions imposed on homosexuality have the effect of reinforcing the status of heterosexuality as the desirable *norm*.

The words 'norm' and 'normal' are heavily loaded in any discussion of sex and sexuality – psychologists and social scientists agree that most individuals want very much to be sexually 'normal' (Tiefer 1995; Strong *et al.* 1996) – so it is important to clarify what they mean.

What is normal?

In terms of sexuality, 'normality' is generally defined in one of four ways: subjective/psychological, conventional/cultural, statistical and biological.

1 Subjective/psychological: This is probably the yardstick that many people use without thinking about it. If something feels normal to us, or if behaving in a particular way leads to feelings of well-being, then we instinctively feel that it is normal. If something feels wrong, or if it causes us to feel guilty, anxious or uncomfortable, then it may feel abnormal. This kind of definition is heavily influenced by socialisation, and may therefore include beliefs about what is morally right or wrong.
2 Conventional/cultural: This refers to the set of values and beliefs about sex and sexuality that are shared within a particular culture. Customs and conventions such as courting rituals, coming-of-age ceremonies and marriage etiquette encourage specific sexual behaviours and discourage others. Sometimes such conventions are supported by legal sanctions, with certain acts forbidden by law. Major social institutions, such as Churches, governments and schools, also play a part in establishing and maintaining them.
3 Statistical: In strictly statistical terms, normal behaviour is simply that which takes place most often within a particular group. This may some-times conflict with other ways of defining normality, since common behaviours are not always conventionally acceptable or 'natural' (see next definition). Thus, although it is not 'natural' for mammals to

coffee, most adults in Britain do so regularly, making it statistically normal. Similarly, although many would argue that it is 'normal' to stay in love with one person throughout a lifetime (in the sense of being socially desirable), this experience is nowadays relatively uncommon and so no longer statistically normal.

4 Biological: Appeals to biological definitions of normality may take three forms: beliefs about what is 'natural' behaviour among animals, beliefs about what is clinically 'normal' in the sense of non-pathological, and beliefs about what is physically normal in the sense of the human biology of reproduction. To judge human behaviour by comparison with animal behaviour is not useful, since we are not comparing like with like. Animals lack our capacity for reason, for fantasy and for conscious choice, for example. Clinical normality in sexuality is also hotly contested. When clinical definitions of normality depart from the purely statistical, they tend to be strongly influenced by convention and morality. Finally, physiological 'normality' is of very little use in establishing norms of behaviour. Our biology equips us to be omnivorous, yet many people choose to live as vegetarians. Similarly, women's biology equips them to produce a child a year throughout their adult life, yet such behaviour is no longer considered normal in Britain.

When social scientists talk about norms and normality, they are generally referring to the second kind of definition; those ideas and values which are shared throughout a particular cultural or social group. Such ideas and values are interesting in themselves, but they also influence the other three measurements of normality. For example, a behaviour that is socially accepted as right and proper is likely to be more widely practised than one which is not. In turn, this will influence which behaviours are commoner than others, and hence which are statistically 'normal' and 'abnormal'. Similarly, our feelings about what is psychologically or subjectively normal are shaped by our socialisation and by the values and beliefs we have been taught. It may appear that biology is entirely separate from culture and convention, yet, as one team of sexologists comments, 'when it comes to specific behaviours, what is biologically normal is what culture defines as normal' (Strong *et al.* 1996: 31).

Sociologists often refer to 'normative' ideas and beliefs. To call an idea or a behaviour 'normative' is to suggest that it has acquired the status of social norm, reinforced by social sanctions. The judgements that establish these normative standards are referred to as 'normalising'; that is, they seek to establish a socially shared notion of normality. In terms of sexuality, the notion of *naturalness* is often called on to support these normalising judgements, as Carabine (1996: 61) explains:

> In relation to sexuality, the normalising effect means that we commonly believe sexuality to be an inherently natural biological drive and that the natural and normal direction of the drive is heterosexual . . . The normalising effect is a means by which appropriate and acceptable sexuality . . . is enforced and regulated.

The idea that an acceptable sexuality may be enforced and regulated is at odds with the widely held belief that sexual feelings and behaviours are instinctive or biologically driven. Most people would probably say that notions of enforcement and regulation have very little to do with their personal experiences of sex and sexuality. In this context, enforcement and regulation do not mean physical or legislative coercion. Rather they refer to *social processes*, some of which involve conscious decisions on the part of policy makers (for example, laws governing the age of consent), but most of which seem to involve little in the way of conscious planning on anyone's part. For example, it is unlikely that any formally established body ever decreed that the question 'Would you like to come back to my place for coffee?' should form part of British courtship rituals, yet, in certain circumstances, the offer of coffee is understood by both parties to be an invitation to participate in sexual contact rather than to share a hot beverage!

Sexual norms and social sanctions

Most members of British society share the conventional belief that hetero-sexuality is normal. Behaviours that do not conform to such social norms are called *deviant* behaviours. In its social scientific usage, 'deviance' does not carry the negative connotations that it has in everyday life; it is simply behaviour which deviates from a social norm. Using this definition it is deviant to own a Rolls Royce or to be an opera singer, since these are not statistically normal behaviours.

Norms that are generally thought to be significant are reinforced by a system of sanctions. Such sanctions may be positive (rewards) and negative (punishments). For example, society values opera singers, so good ones are rewarded with the positive sanctions of fame and high fees to encourage them to continue with their deviant behaviour. On the other hand, society does not value murderers, so they are punished with negative sanctions in the form of lengthy prison sentences to encourage them to cease their deviant behaviours. The positive and negative sanctions that reinforce social norms are also closely tied up with questions of power and status; we can all recall legal scandals where the powerful or privileged have apparently 'got away with murder' because of their position.

Norms and sanctions are also tied up with *authority*. Contemporary social organisation tends to be extremely complex, and we rely on author-itative bodies to state and enforce our norms and values (Ham 1992; Giddens 1997). In the UK such authoritative bodies include the elected government, religious leaders and some professional groups, such as legal experts and members of the medical profession. With the growth in secularism and the increasing status of science since the eighteenth century, the medical profession in particular has acquired considerable authority, and its pronouncements about what is and what is not acceptable human behaviour are taken very seriously indeed (Turner 1995). It is for this reason that the 'medicalisation' of sexuality, discussed later in this book (see p. 59), is of such concern.

Images of sexuality

It is not only authoritative bodies, however, who establish and reinforce normative values. Nor do such values remain constant. Rather, they may be established, reinforced, challenged or changed, and this process goes on ceaselessly. It is part of the living energy of societies and involves the press, media, popular culture, 'high' culture, commerce and new electronic media such as the internet, as well as more formal sectors such as academic research.

By studying these aspects of culture, it is possible to understand how the normative status of heterosexuality is occasionally challenged (by such events as the appearance of sympathetic gay characters in television drama or the success of openly gay pop stars) and also how it is reinforced. It is an interesting exercise to spend a week examining popular culture to assess what proportion of the output reflects lifestyles that do not conform to the heterosexual norm.

Try counting images of heterosexuality, whether overt (as typified in television adverts for certain brands of gravy powder or instant coffee) or covert (for example, in adverts that simply show men and women together in a way which implies the possibility of intimacy). Compare this with the number of references to lesbians or gay men. Films, television programmes, music videos and the lyrics to pop songs or great operas, magazine articles and adverts, television adverts, romantic novels; even illustrations in the *Yellow Pages*® or on the packaging used for breakfast cereals or children's toys, are all sources. Sociologists have long recognised the power of such images to contribute to the cultural construction of shared 'reality', to the extent that they may refer to the stereotypical nuclear family as the 'cereal packet family' (Abercrombie *et al.* 1994).

Such images do not simply reflect what goes on in society. Rather, they *reinforce* social acceptability, and a shared sense of what is normal. In this way the images themselves help to create and reinforce social norms, exerting a powerful influence on our perceptions of reality. This recognition has led to 'positive images' campaigns being launched by black groups, disability rights activists and other marginalised communities in an attempt to redress the balance.

The personal consequences of invisibility

Many heterosexuals are so accustomed to this continual stream of words and images that it may seem trivial. This is not the case for lesbians and gay men. Reading accounts taken from surveys and interviews, or in published autobiographies, it becomes clear that one very significant and hurtful aspect of being lesbian or gay, in the UK and around the world, is this cultural invisibility of lesbian or gay lives (Bradstock and Wakeling 1987; Hall Carpenter Archives 1989; Trenchard 1989; National Lesbian and Gay Survey 1992). The absence of a lesbian or gay 'reflection' in mainstream culture is damaging to the self-esteem of individuals, and makes it hard to feel any sense of belonging in a society which seems not to recognise that you exist. The lack of respectful and positive images can be especially troubling to young people trying to make sense of who they are. Many who grew up at a time when positive images of lesbian or gay life were non-existent, speak movingly of their bewilderment. With no words or images to help them, they simply did not know how to make sense of their experiences; many recall believing that they were the only one in the world with such feelings:

> I thought I was the only person in the world who loved her own sex. Even at seven I suspected my feelings were unusual.
> (Helen: National Lesbian and Gay Survey 1992: 1)

> In our school the anti-sex business was so colossal that almost every-thing was successfully tabooed . . . I didn't regard myself as a homo-sexual, I never thought of this word, nobody knew such a word.
> (David: Porter and Weeks 1991: 42)

> I spent most of my time outside of school alone in my room, secluded from a world that I thought hated me. I was sure of this because I hated myself. I hated being different. I hated myself for being alone.
> (Rhonda: Holmes 1988: 44)

> I was labelled a lesbian by my peers, a charge I denied. Then I asked what a lesbian was, and was referred to the dictionary, but was none the wiser on reading 'a native of the isle of Lesbos'.
> (Vienna: Bradstock and Wakeling 1987: 200)

This cultural silence about the existence of lesbians and gay men was painful for these youngsters, because it was clear to them that the silence was associated with shame and disapproval. The refusal to mention such things gave the very clear message that they were too horrifying even to put into words. Remember Symmonds writing that he could 'hardly find a name [for homosexuality] that will not seem to soil this paper'.

Historically, the long-standing silence about lesbian and gay lives seems to have been, at least in part, motivated by a quite deliberate attempt to re-press homosexuality. When Radclyffe Hall's famous novel about a lesbian, *The Well of Loneliness*, was published in 1927 she stood trial for obscenity. The judge at the trial commented that he would sooner give his children prussic acid to drink than allow them to read Hall's novel (O'Rourke 1989).

The media silence about homosexuality has gradually been eroded, but images of lesbians and gay men were almost unknown in Britain right up to the mid-1980s. And of course it takes more than a few gay-friendly soap operas to compensate for this, as lesbian Ida Burt made clear:

> I get tired of living in a society that acts as though lesbians don't exist, or are invisible, a society in which every visual image, every joke, every nuance of language, suggests that the only normal couple is one composed of a male and a female, and that what every woman

wants is a man. If I had a magic wand I would turn the world around, just for a while, so that being gay was the norm . . . all those sexy ads would feature gay couples, and perhaps there would be one or two well-behaved token non-gays in the all-gay soaps.

(Bradstock and Wakeling 1987: 85)

The invisibility of lesbian and gay lives, combined with the very public visibility of heterosexual lifestyles and behaviours, functions as a mechanism of *social exclusion*. It is significant because media representations have a strong impact on social and cultural norms. Research has shown that heterosexuals are more likely to have positive and accepting attitudes to homosexuality if they have personal contact with a lesbian or gay individual (Pharr 1988; Comstock 1991). On the other hand, individuals who depend on the media for their source of information about homosexuality are more likely to be homophobic.

Reasons and responses

It is important to remember that the sanctions against homosexuality go beyond media invisibility. Same-sex activities and relationships are either prohibited by law or legally discriminated against in almost every country in the world. It seems illogical to make a crime out of an activity that victimises nobody, and to expend scarce police resources on arresting those involved. But this illustrates how difficult it is for many human societies to deal with sex and sexuality. Uninhibited sexual expression seems to be widely regarded as dangerous or threatening to social order, and this is particularly so in complex industrial societies. Sexual behaviour therefore tends to be policed with rigour.

Early theorists, such as Willhelm Reich or Sigmund Freud, suggested that this is because the sexual instinct is a powerful and irresistible force, which has an in-built tendency to work against social stability. According to this kind of model, civilisation itself depends on bringing sexuality firmly under control and repressing sexual drives. More recent thinkers, particularly Michel Foucault, have put forward the idea that, far from being repressed, sex and sexuality are talked about, written about and thought about more than any other aspect of human life (Foucault 1976). According to Foucault, sexuality has not been simply repressed, but rather tends to be manipulated and controlled by those in power.

Consequences: sexual minorities and their subcultures

Academics continue to debate whether the policing of sexual expression is a form of simple repression, or whether Foucault is right in seeing sexuality as one of the instruments of political power. These theoretical debates may appear to have very little to do with 'real life'. Yet the vexed questions of 'normality' versus 'abnormality' and of acceptable behaviour versus unacceptable behaviour have very real consequences for the individuals involved. If you are unlucky enough to have the 'wrong' kind of sexuality this may be enough to lead to you being arrested, imprisoned, humiliated, ostracised or assaulted. You may face rejection from your family or friends, losing your job, being denied any contact with your children or being thrown out of your home. The consequences of the public response to what we generally think of as our most private behaviour can be catastrophic. So how do those whose sexual feelings do not fit into the dominant norm respond to the risks and hostility that they face?

One answer is that, to a greater or lesser degree, they form *subcultures*. Sociologists define a subculture as 'a system of values, attitudes, modes of behaviour and life-styles of a social group which is distinct from, but related to, the dominant culture of society' (Abercrombie *et al.* 1988: 245). Much work has gone into studying such phenomena as the 'youth subculture', or the 'criminal subculture', and subcultures have tended to be associated with deviance. More recently, there has been interest in the relationship between subcultures and market forces.

In the case of certain subcultures, the development of an associated consumer group demanding specific products has led to the growth of particular segments of the commercial market, sometimes known as 'market niches'. But the relationship between subcultures and commercial market niches is not straightforward. Sometimes subcultures develop their own markets, and sometimes existing commercial interests recognise the marketing potential of a subcultural group with disposable income, for example the so-called 'pink economy' in the case of gay men. Some subcultures appear to have been entirely *created* by commercial marketing, as seen in the marketing strategies of the popular music industry, with its sophisticated targeting of age-groups and 'urban tribes'.

In the case of sexual minorities, the formation of a subculture does not always include the formation of a subcultural market. The extent to which a group of people, united only by shared sexual preference, is able to develop a subculture depends to a great extent on the degree to which their sexuality is stigmatised and punished. The autobiographical accounts of gay men and lesbians living under the shadow of criminal law – either those living in Europe or America before decriminalisation or those living today in countries where homosexuality is still illegal – make it very clear that establishing any kind of subculture under such circumstances is extraordinarily difficult. When writing an autobiographical account of the circumstances that led to his trial and imprisonment for homosexuality in 1954, Peter Wildeblood described the life of British gay men at that time as secretive and claustrophobic:

> The homosexual world is, of necessity, compact and isolated. It is also extraordinarily out of touch with reality . . . Our [legal] case caused a momentary flutter, and a number of the better-known homosexuals left the country for a time, until they decided that it was safe to return . . . Their secretiveness and cynicism are imposed on them by the law as it now stands.
>
> (Wildeblood 1955: 184)

With the partial decriminalisation of homosexuality and the commercialisation of post-war culture, a 'gay scene' developed. Here gay men and lesbians were and are able to access the sorts of products and services that mainstream culture takes for granted. It is possible to relax in a pub or cafe (without the constant fear that a homophobic manager will refuse you admission), to buy lesbian- or gay-themed books, cards, videos or calendars (not provided by mainstream publishers and often not stocked by highstreet shops), to behave affectionately towards your partner (without being insulted or attacked), or to get advice about legal, financial or health matters from professionals who are well-informed about the often complex implications of not fitting the norm.

If you live in a world that regards your most intimate relationships as embarrassing, sinful, funny, pitiable, disgusting or wrong, the support offered by a well-established subcultural community is highly important to emotional, psychological and social well-being. It also enables the development of what Foucault called a 'reverse discourse', whereby the tables are turned on the meanings of the dominant culture. For example, confronted with the widely held belief that gay men are effeminate, many gay male communities have actively embraced an extreme form of masculinity. However, the most radical form of reverse discourse among the lesbian and gay community has probably been the assertion that, rather than being a rather sad kind of personal defect, lesbian and gay sexuality can be just as life-enhancing, healthy and mature as heterosexuality.

The ability to develop and participate in a strong subculture is an important strategy for individuals who need to survive the psychological pressures of homophobia. Yet it is not a strategy available to everyone. The lesbian, gay and bisexual community may appear to be vibrant and confident, but it is almost exclusively confined to towns and cities large enough to support a substantial lesbian and gay population. Those living in small towns or rural areas lack the population density or the material resources to form adequately supportive communities, and there is a recognisable gay 'population drift' into larger connurbations in consequence, sometimes referred to in the literature as the 'gay diaspora' (Bell and Valentine 1995). However, not all lesbians or gay men are in a position to be able to migrate, and their isolation in rural areas may be profound. Kramer writes (1995: 211):

> Because of [the] lack of accurate information about homosexuality in nonmetropolitan areas, it may . . . be the case that nonmetropolitan gay men and lesbian women internalise to a greater degree the stigmatising values of the dominant culture, thereby intensifying the internal dissonance all homosexuals feel during the process of personal identity synthesis.

Nor can we assume that *all* urban lesbians and gay men are able to draw on the support of a community. Older people, who grew up under the enforced secrecy of the earlier part of the twentieth century, often find the urban 'scene' alien and geared to younger people. After a lifetime of fear and guilt, older lesbians and gay men may find it extremely hard to trust the new climate of relative openness, and many remain isolated (Macdonald with Rich 1985; Porter and Weeks 1991; Neild and Pearson 1992; Plummer 1995). Racism may effectively exclude many Black lesbians and gay men, the dominance of gay men can alienate many lesbians, the atmosphere of conspicuous consumption can offend those with precious little disposable income, and an emphasis on the 'body beautiful' and on confident sexual display often marginalises disabled lesbians and gay men (see, for example, essays in Kaufmann and Lincoln 1991). Although this subculture offers invaluable support, its resources are sorely stretched, and the support it offers has inevitable restrictions.

Conclusion

We have seen that the social organisation of sex, gender and sexuality is complex, and that it is difficult to unpick the threads of which it consists. It is also clear that issues of power and authority are highly significant. The stigma attached to homosexuality in cultures where heterosexuality retains its normative status has important consequences for individuals and for the policing of sexuality more generally. Far from merely reflecting what goes on in society, cultural representations of sexuality act powerfully to reinforce or to challenge dominant social norms. Although lesbians and gay men have been able to form supportive subcultures, with varying degrees of commercialisation, such subcultures are as fragmented by racism, sexism and ageism as the wider culture, and may have little to offer to those who are not young, white and relatively affluent.

This simplified account of the complex factors which shape the lives of all of us makes it clear that being lesbian or gay may carry heavy costs in terms of personal and social well-being. It suggests that homophobia is likely to be a significant factor in the health and life chances of many individuals, and that sexual orientation is an important human rights issue. The growing recognition that this is so offers a supportive climate to health and social care practitioners wishing to improve their practice in this area.

exercise

Collect a number of recent mainstream magazines and newspapers. Look through them carefully, and take note of any articles that deal with lesbian or gay issues specifically. How many such articles are there? How do they represent homosexuality? Now count the number of illustrations showing couples; include advertisements. How many of these show opposite-sex couples? How many show same-sex couples? Be realistic – do not try to 'force' images into a category they do not in fact fit!

For heterosexual readers

Now obtain a few copies of gay publications (examples include *Diva, Gay Times, The Pink Paper*). Look through carefully, and think about the following questions: How easy was it for you to get hold of these publications? How did you feel about looking for them? Is there anything about them that surprises you?

For lesbian, gay and bisexual readers

Obtain a few copies of gay publications and look through them carefully. How do you think your heterosexual colleagues might react to the contents of these magazines? How does this make you feel? What conclusions can you draw about the impact of your own sexual orientation on your health and well-being?

For all readers

Obtain a copy of *Diva* and a copy of *Cosmopolitan, Marie Claire* or similar glossy woman's magazine. Compare the articles. In particular, compare the amount of space given to articles about sex. What similarities and differences are there? What conclusions might you draw?

Further reading

Comstock, G.D. (1991) *Violence against Lesbians and Gay Men*. New York: Columbia University Press.

Cruikshank, M. (1992) *The Gay and Lesbian Liberation Movement*. London: Routledge.

Deitcher, D. (ed.) (1995) *Over the Rainbow: Lesbian and Gay Politics in America since Stonewall*. London: Boxtree/Channel 4.

Healey, E. and Mason, A. (eds) (1994) *Stonewall 25: The Making of the Lesbian and Gay Community in Britain*. London: Virago.

Mason, A. and Palmer, A. (1996) *Queer Bashing: A National Survey of Hate Crimes Against Lesbians and Gay Men*. London: Stonewall.

Rosenbloom, R. (1996) *Unspoken Rules: Sexual Orientation and Women's Human Rights*. London: Cassell.

Tiefer, L. (1995) *Sex is not a Natural Act and other Essays*. Oxford: Westview Press.

Weeks, J. (1990) *Coming Out: Homosexual Politics in Britain from the Nineteenth Century to the Present*. London: Quartet.

3 a history of ideas about sexuality: culture and religion

Introduction

This chapter gives a brief history of the changing ways in which sexuality has been conceptualised in European culture since the time of the ancient Greeks, and focuses particularly on the role of religion. Aspects of the role of fundamentalism in the modern world are discussed, and the importance of different interpretations of religious texts is stressed. This is followed by a discussion of the impact of religious intolerance on lesbian, gay and bisexual communities and individuals, and the chapter concludes by examining some of the ways in which those communities and individuals have responded.

What do history and theology have to do with practice?

Famously, the three topics of conversation to be avoided at the polite dinner party are sex, religion and politics. All can arouse strong passions and vigorous argument, and a person's sex life and religious belief are both generally regarded as private. History, on the other hand, is often thought of as boring and irrelevant. Yet there are compelling reasons for underpinning any exploration of the sociology of sexualities with a basic understanding of both history and theology.

We are, as Peter Hamilton notes, 'almost programmed into thinking of our sexuality as a wholly natural feature of life' (cited in Weeks 1985: 7). Because of this, it can be difficult, even threatening, to take a mental 'step back' and examine our own beliefs about sexuality. Perhaps this is especially true for nurses and other health care professionals, whose training depends on the medical model of health and well-being. This model is based on the belief that there are healthy bodies and unhealthy bodies, normal functions and abnormal functions, and that it is the job of medicine to eradicate the unhealthy and abnormal. Similarly, the social care professions lay great emphasis on notions of functionality and dysfunctionality and of family stability. It is easy to see that there is likely to be 'slippage' between these ideas and questions of morality, and this has often been the case with questions of sex and sexuality.

Studying the history of changing ideas about sexuality is useful for two reasons. First, it enables us to look objectively at our own beliefs and may help us respect those of others. Second, it can help us to work out where our own beliefs come from, why we hold them, and to what extent they influence our work. This reflexivity is absolutely central to professionalism in health and social care since, without it, we may be more concerned to 'protect' our sense of what is right than to safeguard the integrity of our client. So understanding what the ancient Greeks thought about sex, or what different religions say about homosexuality, is surprisingly relevant to the professional practice of those who care for others.

There is a widely held belief that ancient Greek society was the cradle of European civilisation. Since huge areas of the planet were subsequently colonised by Europeans, it is likely that the social organisation of sexuality in many parts of the world will owe something to European thinking about sex, and this, too, suggests that we should understand something of this distant history.

The ideas of the ancient Greeks belong to history, but religion remains a vital component of contemporary life for many. Indeed, the holistic definition of health championed by the World Health Organization (WHO) includes spiritual health and well-being. There is also evidence that HSC practitioners with strong religious beliefs are more likely to hold negative attitudes to their lesbian or gay clients (Shernoff and Scott 1988; Stevens 1993). It is, therefore, also important to have some understanding of current religious debates on sexuality.

Some insight into the politics of religion is also important. With colonialism came the religious doctrines of the invaders, so that Judaeo-

Christianity and Islam, together with their teachings about human sexual morality, spread to the areas controlled by European or Muslim invaders (Smart 1989). An important characteristic of our own postmodern world is the rise of fundamentalist movements, whether Islamic, Christian, Hindu or Sikh, and such movements may have a dramatic impact on the sexual cultures under their influence.

Ancient Greece

Many assume that the ancient Greeks were tolerant of homosexuality; indeed, Victorian and early twentieth-century writers often refer to same-sex love as 'Greek love'. This assumption is understandable, given that many of the most important historical figures from ancient Greece seem to fit a contemporary definition of homosexuality. Philosophers such as Plato and Aristotle, heroic conquerors such as Alexander the Great or great writers such as Sappho all seem to have been openly and unashamedly the lovers of members of their own sex. This seemed an anomaly to the Victorians, who revered classical Greek culture as much as they loathed homosexuality. Symonds expresses this confusion when he refers to homo-sexuality as 'a problem in Greek ethics' (Symonds 1984: 9).

However, historians now believe that it is a misunderstanding to think of the ancient Greeks as being tolerant of homosexuality in the same way as a modern society, such as Sweden or the Netherlands. This is partly because the very idea of a homosexual as a specific type of person is historically recent, and unknown to Greeks of the classical era. They could not have been tolerant of homosexuality any more than they could have expressed an opinion on traffic lights. To imagine that they were is, in the literal meaning of the word, anachronistic – taking things out of their historical context. The 'problem in Greek ethics' is a problem for Symonds the Victorian, not for the ancient Greeks.

Classical Greek society was very hierarchical. Although it was the first ever democracy, the body of people eligible to vote and to run the country were a small and select group. You could only vote, or be a fully func-tioning member of Greek society, if you were a free adult male citizen, not a boy, a woman, a slave or a foreigner. And, as is so often the case, the power relationships of Greek sexual culture mirrored those of Greek political life. The primary sexual division seems not to have been between women and men, but between adult, male, Greek citizens and every-body else.

An adult, male, Greek citizen had the right to choose as their sexual partner anyone from the other side of this divide, and would be expected to be the 'active' partner in any sexual acts with that other person. To penetrate women, boys, slaves or foreigners with your penis was a mark of your proper status. To *be* penetrated was shameful (Halperin 1989), but otherwise it seems to have mattered very little whether your taste ran to male or female partners, although it might lead to teasing if your preferences were particularly strong.

Once this is understood it is easier to make sense of the fact that the Greeks lacked the concept 'homosexuality' altogether. We divide people up into homosexual, heterosexual and bisexual because these divisions seem very important to us, but they were far less so to the ancient Greeks. We have also learnt to regard homosexuals and heterosexuals as entirely different *types of person*, so much so that we are able to ask what 'causes homosexuality'. Our interest in this question is quite genuine, but to an ancient Greek it would be rather like asking what 'causes' someone to prefer heavy metal music to hip hop.

It is clear, then, that the ancient Greeks regarded what we call sexual orientation more as a matter of personal taste than as a defining characteristic of personal identity. Understanding this takes us on to the next stage of our enquiry. If the ancient Greeks thought that sexual orientation was simply a matter of taste, and contemporary Europeans believe something so dramatically different, this changes the kinds of question we must ask. Instead of asking 'what makes someone gay or straight' we need to ask, 'what makes us think that either "gay" or "straight" is something you can *be* at all?' And how did this come to be seen as such an important aspect of human behaviour that, in some parts of the world, it justifies imprisonment, social exclusion or even the death penalty? There are, as we shall see, no easy answers.

Religion and sex

Religious belief plays an important part in shaping cultural attitudes to sex and the social organisation of sexuality. Social historians and anthropologists tell us that there have been and still are many cultures that accept some forms of same-sex love, or which permit biological men to live as if they were women and vice versa (Caplan 1987; Bremmer 1989; Duberman *et al.* 1989; Epstein and Straub 1991; Ramet 1996). Indeed, the behaviours that we call 'homosexual' seem to be regarded as ordinary in the majority of cultures studied by anthropologists (Webb 1985).

In many such cultures there exists a religious or spiritual interpretation of these behaviours. For example, some native American tribes recognised the existence of 'two-spirit' people, individuals whose spirit guides required them to live as if they were a member of the other sex. Although such individuals appear to have been teased, it was clearly accepted that they should live out the role of the opposite sex, including sexually (Califia 1997). Catholic French colonial invaders, coming from a very different spiritual tradition, were shocked by the cultural acceptance of these two-spirit people, whom they called 'berdaches' (Whitehead 1993).

Although some religious and spiritual traditions accept the diversity of human sexuality, others are more rigid. In many parts of the world, religious teaching is used to justify human rights abuses against lesbians, gay men and others who transgress sexual protocols (Clark 1994; Lee *et al.* 1995; Rosenblum 1996; Vincent 1996). Yet there is controversy, even within the traditions themselves, about the morality of such abuses.

It is important to distinguish here between religion and fundamentalism, since it is clearly possible to hold strong religious beliefs and remain tolerant of sexual diversity. Indeed, many lesbians, gay men and bisexuals are active members of their own religious cultures and strive to integrate their sexuality and their faith (Stuart 1992; Helminiak 1994; Vincent 1996).

Fundamentalism

Fundamentalists not only hold strong personal beliefs but insist that everyone else should obey the teachings of their particular religion. Fundamentalism means something very specific; the belief that religion and politics are the same thing, that the state should be run according to religious law, and that the judicial system should enforce obedience to a particular creed (Sahgal and Yuval-Davis 1992; Reinfelder 1995). Unbelievers or heretics may be excluded from the state, punished or killed, since fundamentalism admits of no debate or religious tolerance. One British coalition from different religious traditions defines fundamentalism as 'modern political movements which use religion as the basis for mobilisation in an attempt to win or consolidate power and exercise social control' (Bard and Cummins 1995: 1)

Iran is a clear example of a fundamentalist Muslim state, and as such is regarded with great anxiety by the secular societies of the West. Recent years have witnessed the spread of terrorism by some fundamentalist Muslim groups, paralleled by the growth of what some commentators refer to as 'Islamophobia' in the West (Clark 1994: 10; Pieterse 1994). But neither fundamentalism nor fundamentalist terrorism are restricted to Islam. It is, after all, right-wing Christian fundamentalists who are responsible for the anti-choice campaigns in the US that involve bombing abortion clinics and shooting doctors who perform terminations, whilst Hindu, Muslim and Sikh fundamentalists have all been involved in violence and terrorist activities in India and Pakistan.

Historically, many European nations were governed on fundamentalist principles, including the UK. The monarch to this day holds the title 'defender of the faith', although religious law no longer controls government. Throughout those periods in European history when religious law did underpin state government, homosexual behaviour was often severely punished, and the death penalty was not uncommon (Duberman *et al.* 1989). One important consequence of European colonial invasions was that religious law based on Christian doctrine was subsequently imposed on the conquered nations. Historian Jonathan Katz has documented the implications of this for the treatment of lesbians and gay men in the United States (Katz 1983), noting that homosexual behaviour among European settlers was regarded as sinful and was severely punished, often by death.

Although such attitudes no longer control government and legal process in the US, religious fundamentalism remains an important and influential part of American life. There are powerful and wealthy groups who explicitly target sexual and gender behaviours; abortion, women's rights and gay rights feature prominently as aspects of contemporary American society which they are dedicated to overthrowing.

As mainstream sociology has long recognised, 'Virtually all major religions encourage male dominance' (Macionis and Plummer 1997). So it is perhaps not surprising that fundamentalist Christian groups promote a form of social organisation where women's purpose in life is to be wives and mothers, where sexual behaviour is only permissible within the context of a procreative marriage, and where abortion and same-sex relationships are prohibited. In this, they have much in common with some Islamic fundamentalists (Mernissi 1986).

Fundamentalists, of whatever religion, take their authority from scriptural teaching. Yet the existence of many denominations, factions and schisms within the major religions point to the existence of debate – even conflict – about the interpretation of such teachings. Within the Jewish faith, for example, attitudes to homosexuality vary from the liberal to the hostile. Whilst Reform Judaism routinely ordains lesbian or gay rabbis, Orthodox and Hasidic Jews remain intolerant (Macionis and Plummer 1997).

What does the Bible say about homosexuality?

Since the Bible is so often used to justify negative attitudes towards gay people, it is a useful exercise to examine what it actually says about homosexuality, and to discuss some recent interpretations. The Bible, as used in most Christian denominations, is divided into two parts: the Old Testament, which contains the books of the ancient Jewish prophets, and the New Testament, which contains the Gospels (four separately authored accounts of the life and work of Jesus) and a collection of Epistles (letters) written by St Paul to early Christian communities.

These texts vary in their approach to homosexual acts. There is no mention whatsoever of homosexuality in the Gospels, and hence no support for the view that it is abhorrent (or otherwise) to Jesus Christ. On the other hand, St Paul voiced very negative views (Comstock 1991; Helminiak 1994), to the extent that some modern commentators have suggested – anachronistically – that he was repressing his own homosexual tendencies.

Most Christian fundamentalists base their hostility towards lesbians and gay men on two passages in the Old Testament: Chapter 18, verse 22 in Leviticus and the story of Sodom and Gomorrah in Genesis, the first and most ancient Biblical text. These writings were produced by nomadic tribesmen in ancient times and it is often difficult to apply them effectively to contemporary life in the industrialised West. In addition, they have been translated and retranslated, and this has inevitably resulted in some degree of distortion and misinterpretation.

We have seen that the notion of 'homosexuality' would not have been recognised by the ancient Greeks, and by the same token it would not have made much sense to the tribal societies of the Old Testament Middle East. As Mollenkott points out:

> The word *homosexual* does not occur anywhere in the Bible. No
> extant text, no manuscript, neither Hebrew nor Greek, Syriac nor
> Aramaic, contains the word . . . the use of the word *homosexuality* by
> certain English Bible translators is an example of . . . extreme bias.
>
> (Cited in Pharr 1988: 3)

Moreover, careful historical scholarship has recently unearthed evidence
of Christian same-sex 'marriage ceremonies' dating back to the Middle
Ages (Boswell 1994). Medieval Christians cannot, on this evidence, have
believed that the Bible condemned such unions. This strongly suggests
that the Biblical condemnation of homosexuality springs from an historically recent interpretation, leading one Catholic priest to conclude: 'The
question is not "What are the Bible texts on homosexuality?" . . . The
question is, "How do you interpret these texts?" ' (Helminiak 1994: 21).

Many contemporary biblical scholars now agree that the sin for which
the cities of Sodom and Gomorrah were destroyed is not homosexuality
at all, and that this is a modern Western interpretation, which distorts
the original scriptural text (Pharr 1988; Hasbany 1989; Comstock 1991;
Tannahill 1992; Helminiak 1994). These two 'cities of the plain' are now
thought to have been destroyed for their refusal to offer hospitality to
strangers. In a desert land, where food and water were scarce, hospitality
was often a matter of life and death and was therefore a key element in
the culture of this highly moral society. By refusing hospitality, the citizens
of Sodom and Gomorrah were breaking this most essential rule for desert
living, and it was for this that they were punished (Pharr 1988).

The book of Leviticus, the religious laws governing the tribal peoples of
ancient Israel, states 'Thou shalt not lie with mankind as with womankind.
It is abomination' (Chapter 18, verse 22). There is little room for misinterpretation here. But Leviticus spends far longer dealing with the problem of
leprosy (116 lines, as opposed to the one line devoted to 'homosexuality'),
and other matters such as food hygiene and purification rituals. This
suggests that homoscxuality, although not permitted by these nomadic
societies, was not regarded to be particularly important.

There is also the question of selectivity. Whilst modern Christian
fundamantalists are quick to draw on Leviticus to insist that homosexual
behaviour is an abomination, they tend to be less inclined to propose that
we adhere to the other Levitican rules. These include: that a priest must
cleanse a leper by killing a bird in an earthenware pot and washing
another live bird in its blood; that a menstruating woman must sacrifice
two pigeons seven days aftcr each period and that anyone who curses
their father or mother, or who commits adultery should be put to death.

It is simply not appropriate to adopt such regulations for contemporary
social organisation; there would be an outcry if women started slaughtering
pigeons at the end of each period or if adulterers – including philandering
politicians and presidents – were executed. So why pull this one rule out
of Leviticus and ignore all the rest?

This selectivity has, quite reasonably, lead those arguing for tolerance
within the Christian faith to ask for further justification:

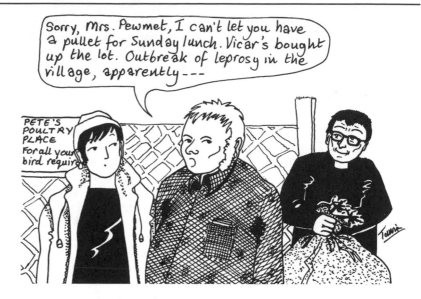

Whatever may be the traditions held in the Judaeo-Christian ethic about homosexuality, we would suggest that those who maintain that homosexual acts are intrinsically wrong are under an obligation to show why the suffering that this causes to so many individuals is necessary . . . what the modern world asks of religious believers who condemn homosexuality is to prove to them that what they are exercising is not just a cultural prejudice.

(Murray and McClure 1995: 42)

None of this is to suggest that 'pro-gay' interpretations of sacred texts are 'right' and anti-gay interpretations are 'wrong'. What it does demonstrate is that any religion based on a holy book is inevitably dependent on human *interpretation* of these ancient texts. And those human interpretations are likely to shift in response to changing social and political circumstances, meaning that there is always debate and sometimes heated conflict. In the end, those who draw on religious texts to justify discrimination against any group have a responsibility to demonstrate that such discrimination has beneficial outcomes in the contemporary context.

Implications for lesbian and gay human rights

Religious fundamentalism in its many forms is behind many abuses of the human and civil rights of lesbians and gay men around the world (Rosenblum 1996; War on Want 1996). Among the most distressing examples of this is the current situation in Iran. Iran is governed by a very

Table 3.1 Sums spent by the religous right in the US

Group	Amount spent per annum	Purpose
Focus on the Family (Colorado)	$150 million	Fighting abortion and gay rights
Christian Coalition (Virginia)	$25 million	Fighting abortion, gay rights, women's rights
Concerned Women for America (Washington)	$14 million	Fighting abortion, gay rights, sex education

Source: Ms, 6(2) (Sept/Oct 1995)

strict form of Islamic law (called the *Sharia*), which considers homosexual behaviour to be 'one of the worst possible sins imaginable'. A judge may order the execution of any individual believed to be lesbian or gay without trial; it is not even necessary for anyone to put a formal complaint to the authorities, and very little evidence is required (Reinfelder 1995; War on Want 1996). Lesbian and gay Iranians live in daily fear for their lives, and several times a year some are publicly executed. Fierce political struggle continues in Iran (Mernissi 1986; Afshar 1994), the outcome of which remains to be seen.

In the United States, right-wing Christian fundamentalism and institutional Catholicism are the most powerful and dedicated opponents of the lesbian and gay movement for civil rights. Christian religious leaders are involved in politics at the highest level (Blasius and Phelan 1997) and fundamentalist groups spend billions of dollars every year on political campaigning.

With such substantial sums of money involved, the religious right has been able to block the passage of laws protecting the civil rights of lesbians, gays and bisexuals in many States of the Union, and to prevent the Clinton administration from fulfilling election promises made to the lesbian and gay community.

The harm done by religious intolerance of homosexuality is not confined to the large-scale level of politics. On a personal level, many devout individuals of every faith face a painful struggle between their religious belief and their own sexual orientation, a struggle that may be devastating to self-esteem and emotional well-being (Helminiak 1994). Even in post-apartheid South Africa, with a new constitution safeguarding lesbian and gay rights, a recent study concluded that, 'It is people from communities where religious or cultural taboos against homosexuality are strongest, who are most vulnerable' (Griffin *et al.* 1998: 12).

In the UK, the most extreme examples of the harm that may be done to individuals in the name of Christianity are to be found in the 'Ex-Gay' ministries, evangelical organisations that claim to be able to 'cure' homosexuality by prayer. Some ex-gay groups state that, 'Those with homosexual feelings are, by definition, not Christians', or that 'Homosexual feelings are the consequence of demon possession' (Green *et al.* 1996: 27). It is not difficult to imagine how a young person, struggling to come to terms with such 'feelings' might react to these teachings. One such young man, recounting his experiences with the Jesus Army, writes that:

> I got headaches frequently while they questioned me and accused me of doing things I had not done . . . After leaving, I had many nightmares about demons and worries of death. I also had problems speaking to other men . . . I used to jump at the sight of my own shadow and I developed a fear of the dark . . . The mind is left confused and obsessed.
>
> (Green *et al.* 1996: 74–75)

Experiences such as this are clearly not conducive to self-esteem and mental well-being.

The community responds

Lesbian, gay and bisexual believers have responded to religious intolerance in three ways. Some have formed activist groups of both believers and non-believers to challenge church teaching; others have worked for increased tolerance or have established their own forms of worship within the established churches; and others have turned away from mainstream religion to develop different forms of spiritual expression. There is also a growing theology of sexuality, which acts as a forum for academic as well as spiritual debate (see, for example, Isherwood and Stuart 1998).

Activism

Just as fundamentalism is principally political in nature, so too is anti-fundamentalist activism. The human rights organisation, Amnesty International, and the development charity, War on Want, are typical of those mainstream groups that have recently recognised the need to end human rights abuses against lesbians and gay men, including those associated with fundamentalism. Activists also campaign in response to specific political situations. In the US, for example, the Stop the Church campaign was initiated by the Aids Coalition to Unleash Power (ACTUP). It carried out demonstrations and 'zaps' in response to Cardinal O'Connor's homophobic response to the HIV pandemic (Blasius and Phelan 1997). In Britain, the lesbian and gay rights activist group, OUTrage, often led by veteran campaigner Peter Tatchell, has demonstrated against the Church of England's refusal to ordain gay clergy, whilst four leaders of an Italian gay rights group sued Pope Paul VI in 1976, claiming that 'their personal dignity had been harmed by the Pope's description of homosexuality as "shameful", "infamous" and "horrible"' (Tannahill 1992: 153).

Working from within

There is ample evidence of a growing desire, within at least some religious traditions, to make reparation for past abuses perpetrated against lesbian and gay people and to foster a new spirit of inclusiveness. For example, the Evangelical Church of Berlin-Brandenburg issued the following statement in August 1991:

> The exclusion of people with a homosexual character has a long and painful prehistory in our society. We regret that the Christian Church also bears a considerable share of the blame. The silence of Christians during the Nazi period about the murder of homosexuals in the concentration camps is one part of this shared guilt.
>
> (Cited in Grau 1995: forematter)

Those for whom religious faith is as important as their sexuality, within whatever religion, are working to develop a new, more compassionate and tolerant faith, which values and welcomes strong, loving relationships, regardless of the gender of the people involved. Some have chosen to set up their own Churches, or to establish support groups within Church communities. Of these, probably the most substantial is the Metropolitan Community Church, which was set up in the US by the Reverend Troy Perry, and now has branches in England. Support groups include the Catholic lesbian and gay group Dignity, the Lesbian and Gay Christian Movement and the Friends Homosexual Fellowship. In the US, the size-able Black gay community have their own Church (Tinney 1996) offering spiritual community to individuals confronting racism as well as homophobia. A further significant intervention in the UK was the publication in 1992 of a lesbian and gay liturgy, *Daring to Speak Love's Name*, whose author looked forward to 'the day when lesbian and gay people are welcomed into all Christian communities and celebrated for who they are' (Stuart 1992: xvii).

Alternative spiritualities

A further response to exclusion from established religions has been for many lesbians and gay men to explore alternative spiritual traditions, or to invent their own. Gay writer, Edmund White, for example, found support in Bhuddism during his painful early years (White 1982, 1997). Others have looked to ancient pre-Christian traditions to provide the building blocks of a version of new age spirituality, which includes a celebration of the erotic and of the magical potential of gender-reversal, and to establish a positive mythography and symbolism for lesbian and gay life (Grahn 1984; Thompson 1987).

For those who are as uneasy with new age philosophies as with established religious tradition, an alternative strategy has been to start building lesbian and gay cultural traditions from the beginning. In the introduction to her collection of lesbian commitment ceremonies, Becky Butler (1990: vii) writes, 'With the arrival of each new account of a ceremony, I have felt as though I were witnessing the creation of new traditions and new paths.'

Conclusion

Religious fundamentalism is a powerful stumbling block for lesbian and gay communities fighting for their civil and human rights, and the apparent conflict between religious belief and a desire to respect the life choices of others is difficult for many individuals. Nevertheless, a shared sense of spirituality is often important to individuals and to communities. This has led, as we have seen, to conflict within religions, to much hostility between lesbian and gay communities and the religious establishments that oppose them, and to much suffering. But there are some encouraging signs of greater acceptance. Ironically, perhaps, some established Churches have found increased compassion and respect for gay communities in response to the HIV pandemic:

> Every year in New York City, there is a Gay Pride March. Because so many people from our communities have died of AIDS, we've built two minutes of silence into this event. Churches throughout the city pay respect to our moment of remembrance and ring their bells in unison.
>
> (Blasius and Phelan 1997: 625)

The struggle for tolerance has hardly begun within Muslim communities or Catholicism, and right-wing fundamentalism remains implacably opposed to gay human and civil rights. Yet, as American Christian activists Robert Nugent and Jeannine Gramick (1989: 43) assert, change may be on the horizon:

> The fishbone [of homophobia] remains caught in the churches' collective throat and will neither be swallowed nor ejected easily or soon. But there are strong and positive signs that serious attempts are underway in all of the mainline denominations to find answers to the questions confronting the believing community.

The 'strong and positive signs' identified by Nugent and Gramick offer powerful support to devout health and social care practitioners who may struggle to reconcile religious belief with professional obligation. For practitioners who are not themselves religious, informed understanding may enable effective support to be offered to service users for whom such questions are extremely significant. The WHO definition of health, after all, encompasses spiritual well-being.

exercise

For heterosexual readers

Spend a few minutes reflecting on what you have learnt in this chapter. You may find it useful to make brief notes of some key points. What do you think lesbian or gay readers might feel about the material discussed in this chapter? Jot down a few sentences about the kinds of thoughts and feelings which they might have. Now imagine yourself discussing this chapter with a colleague who is lesbian or gay. What would you want to say to them? Would you want to ask any questions? If so, write down these questions or anything you would like to discuss with them. Now read what you have written. What does it tell you about yourself? Can you think of anything positive that you could do with this information?

For lesbian or gay readers

Spend a few minutes thinking about what you have read in this chapter. How much of it was new to you? Did you learn anything useful? You may find it helpful to jot down some brief notes. It is likely that most of the people who read this chapter will be heterosexual. What do you think their reactions might be to what they read? What would you *like* their reactions to be? Is there anything *you* would like to say to them about this chapter? If so, write down your comments. Now read through what you have written. What does it tell you about the conditions you work under, as a lesbian or gay man working in health or social care? Can you think of something positive that you can do with this information?

Further reading

Butler, B. (1990) *Ceremonies of the Heart: Celebrating Lesbian Unions*. Washington: Seal Press.

Grahn, J. (1984) *Another Mother Tongue: Gay Words, Gay Worlds*. Boston: Beacon Press.

Hasbany, R. (ed.) (1989) *Homosexuality and Religion*. New York: Harrington Park Press.

Helminiak, D. (1994) *What the Bible Really Says About Homosexuality*. San Francisco: Alamo Square Press.

Isherwood, L. and Stuart, E. (1998) *Introducing Body Theology*. Sheffield: Sheffield Academic Press.

Stuart, E. (1992) *Daring to Speak Love's Name: A Gay and Lesbian Prayer Book*. London: Hamish Hamilton.

Theology and Sexuality, the journal of the Centre for the Study of Christianity and Sexuality. Sheffield: Sheffield Academic Press.

Thompson, M. (1987) *Gay Spirit: Myth and Meaning*. New York: St Martin's Press.

4 science and sexuality: the medical model and its implications

Introduction

Religious interpretations of homosexual behaviour tend to focus on the behaviour, not the individual. The behaviour is a sin, it represents an individual giving in to temptation. There is no notion that sinning or being tempted in this way makes you a specific kind of person, 'a homosexual', it just makes you (in common with everyone else) a sinner. You may repent of your sin and be forgiven, or you may expiate your sin by some ritual of atonement or by your death. In common with the ancient Greeks, such scriptural beliefs do not recognise the existence of 'the homosexual'. To understand where that idea originated, we need to turn to the rise of science and rationalism. This chapter gives a brief overview of scientific thinking on homosexuality, discusses some of the most important current theories and looks at the social and political implications.

Doctor knows best: the rise of rationalism and medical science

Belief in the importance of rational thought began to challenge the dominance of religion during the Enlightenment, an era in European history, which reached its zenith during the eighteenth century. Of course there are no clear-cut boundaries in history, and the dominance of rational thought has waxed and waned over the centuries, often in a close relationship to the coming and going of religious faiths (Porter 1997). Nevertheless, the Enlightenment was a time during which the sciences developed at a dramatic pace and in which new discoveries were made, which led people to believe that nature could be conquered by harnessing the power of experimental science.

Scientists and philosophers began to paint a picture of a world governed, not by invisible demons and an angry god, but by natural forces, which human beings could learn to understand and then to control. For Europeans of the eighteenth and nineteenth centuries (and, indeed, in the early part of the twentieth century), science seemed to hold out the promise of a Utopia where disease and pain were vanquished and all could live in safety and peace.

Science and sex: sexology

Along with the idea that nature had 'laws' which could be understood and controlled, came the idea that so too did human 'nature'. By the end of the nineteenth century, two developing human sciences, psychology and sociology, were attempting to discover the laws governing human behaviour. Psychology concentrated on the internal world of the individual and sociology on the interactions of groups and entire societies. The nineteenth century saw a growing obsession with classification, which led, among other things, to the development of sexology. This new science set out to apply scientific methods to the study of human sexuality. At the same time, the rapidly growing profession of medicine was asserting its own claim to the study of human nature and human behaviour.

As was the case with most scientific enterprise at the cusp of the nineteenth and twentieth centuries, the pioneer sexologists tended to be enthusiastic amateurs trained in a great range of disciplines and included psychiatrists, doctors, poets and political activists. Each had their own theory of homosexuality, and such theories varied widely.

The early sexologists were often either 'gay' themselves or were deeply sympathetic to the unhappiness suffered by their homosexual contemporaries. Whatever the unintended consequences of their work

Table 4.1 Pioneers in sexology

Karl Maria Kertbeny	1824–1882	German, coined the term 'homosexuality' in an article published in 1869 (anonymously).
Karl Heinrich Ulrichs	1825–1895	German, published 12 volumes on homosexuality, which he called 'uranianism'. He himself 'came out' as an 'urning' to a convention of German jurists. Saw 'urnings' as members of a third sex.
Carl von Westphal	1833–1890	German physician, one of the first to study lesbianism, which he termed an example of 'contrary sexual impulse' and believed to be harmless.
Richard von Krafft-Ebing	1840–1902	Austrian, Professor of Psychiatry at the University of Vienna. Published *Psychopathia Sexualis* in 1882, detailing a huge number of sexual 'perversions', including homosexuality, which he attributed to a 'diseased condition of the central nervous system'.
John Addington Symonds	1840–1893	British poet, critic and writer on sexuality. Was himself gay, and wrote *A Problem in Greek Ethics*, about attitudes to homosexuality in classical Greece, and *Sexual Inversion*. His writings were suppressed by his family after his death.
Edward Carpenter	1844–1929	British socialist, vegetarian and feminist sympathiser. Wrote *The Intermediate Sex* in 1908, in which he suggested that same-sex love was a sign of inner androgyny, which he saw as a force for good.
Sigmund Freud	1856–1939	Austrian, the founding father of modern psychology. Believed that all human beings are essentially bisexual, and that exclusive heterosexuality was as much in need of explanation as exclusive homosexuality. Although Freud himself insisted that homosexuality was not dysfunctional, many of his followers promoted the belief that homosexuality was an immature or disturbed form of sexual expression.
Henry Havelock Ellis	1859–1939	British, medically trained. Wrote about homosexuality as 'inversion' and homosexual people as 'inverts'. Sponsored the British Society for the Study of Sex Psychology. His wife, Edith, was a lesbian.
Magnus Hirschfeld	1868–1935	German, early gay rights activist and psychologist. His pioneering work on homosexuality was sparked off by the trials of Oscar Wilde in England, and by the suicide of one of his own gay patients on the eve of his wedding. Founded the Scientific Humanitarian Committee in 1898, and established the Institute for Sexual Science in Berlin. The Institute was disbanded by the Nazis, who raided it and burned Hirschfeld's collection of books and papers.

(some of which are discussed below), their intentions were good. Historian Jeffrey Weeks (1985: 14) reminds us that sexology has been important in 'extending our knowledge of sexual behaviours'. Several among them were medically trained, and this had particularly important implications for modern theories of sexuality. The effect was to replace the idea that homosexuality was a sin with the concept of homosexuality as disease or malfunction. Notions of pathology superseded those of moral failing. Commentators refer to this as the 'pathologisation' or 'medical-isation' of sexuality.

Inversion

The most influential element of modern thinking about sexuality which developed at this time was the notion of *inversion*. This idea was inherited by the sexologists rather than originating with them. Their thinking did not emerge in a vacuum. The early sexologists were all nationals of England, Austria or Germany, countries where the Protestant religious tradition was powerful, and they were all nineteenth-century professional gentlemen. Their 'new' theories were inevitably influenced by this cultural context. Alfred Kinsey was to write that they produced, 'scientific classifica-tions . . . nearly identical with theologic classifications and with moral pronouncements of the English common law of the fifteenth century' (Weeks 1985: 66).

The notion of 'inversion' was based on late nineteenth-century European beliefs about what was 'normal' sexual behaviour for men and women. Heterosexuality, ran the familiar argument, was biologically ordained. Therefore, homosexual desire indicated some form of inversion, or turning upside-down, of sex. This was the thinking behind various early models of homosexuality such as the 'contrary sexual impulse', the 'third sex' and even Edward Carpenter's positive notion of 'androgyny'. This line of thought was to underpin almost all medico-scientific attempts to under-stand homosexuality right up to our own times, including those of Freud and his followers (Ruse 1988).

Science and more science: some current developments

At the dawn of the twenty-first century, more research money is being spent on trying to explain same-sex love and desire than at any time in history. There are three competing theories which claim to have established a biological cause for homosexuality: one suggests that it is sparked off *in utero* by hormonal accident; another that it results from atypical brain structure; and the third that it is the consequence of genetic predisposition. All three theories contain elements of the Victorian notion of inversion.

In the early decades of the twentieth century, theories linking homo-sexuality to gender inversion led researchers down some rather muddy avenues. Lacking the technology to probe the cell biology and chemical reactions of neurones, hormones and chromosomes, they concentrated on examining those large-scale characteristics of the body visible to the naked eye. In New York, the Committee for the Study of Sex Variance (CSSV) spent six years (from 1935 to 1941) carrying out detailed examination of the genitals of 'sex variant' men and women, in order to identify the characteristics of 'sex variant genitalia'.

Researchers, led by gynaecologist Robert Dickinson, drew composite sketches of the 'sex variant pelvis' (merging the measurements obtained from both gay men and lesbians) and oddities such as the 'typical sex variant vulva', which were published in book form in 1941. Dickinson and his colleagues drew the conclusion that everything about female sex variant genitals was bigger than that of normal women, with the exception of the uterus, which he claimed was small. In particular he drew attention to the 'notably erectile' clitoris (Terry 1995: 143).

The researchers in the sex variant study were motivated by the assumption that lesbian sexuality was *more like* heterosexual masculine sexuality than heterosexual female sexuality. Because masculine sexuality was thought to be stronger and more urgent than female sexuality, and to be primarily concerned with a drive to penetrate, lesbians were assumed to have a rudimentary penis (the 'notably erectile' clitoris), and simply possessed a larger version of everything else – vulva, vagina, hymen, even nipples – than their less lusty 'normal' sisters.

Proper female sexuality was at this time assumed to be driven by a deep longing for children rather than by desire for gratification (Hubback 1957), so the sex variant woman would, naturally, have a smaller uterus. A small body part was associated with a weak drive (in this case, towards reproduction), whilst large body parts were associated with strong drives (here, towards sexual gratification). The logic was analogous to believing that people with big mouths would be more interested in food than those with small mouths, or that individuals with large feet might enjoy dancing more than those with small feet.

Similar assumptions led to claims that you could distinguish lesbians from normal women by their fondness for male activities such as smoking, their (unnatural) ability to whistle, or their interest in unwomanly pursuits such as science or politics (Showalter 1987; Ruse 1988; Wilton 1995). In a similar drive to prove that gay men were effeminate, researchers laboriously measured factors such as strength of grip and body mass (Ruse 1988), whilst others claimed that the typical gay man's penis was 'underdeveloped, tapered . . . resembling that of a dog' and that his anus was 'naturally smooth, lacking in radial folds' (cited in Haeberle 1989).

Scientific rationality?

Such accounts now seem misguided, yet they remain important for two reasons. First, they illustrate what may happen when a concern to 'explain homosexuality' – rather than a more open-ended question – drives research. Second, they point to the immense credibility of medical science, and the often uncritical way in which its 'findings' are received. None of the assertions about lesbian and gay bodies made by experts in the 1940s and 1950s was based on empirical evidence or rigorous scientific method. The researchers had made up their minds about what they were going to find *before* carrying out their enquiries, and routinely manipulated their findings in order to fit their predetermined narratives (Terry 1995). Yet, *because they are scientists*, their work is presented as scientific fact and is readily accepted as such, sometimes by clinical practitioners as well as by lay people. For example, the myth of the super-large lesbian clitoris persisted well into the 1970s, as Barale comments:

> Frank Caprio, M.D., states not only that some lesbians have 'an unusually elongated clitoris' but provides the datum of 'about six centimetres', while the ever knowledgeable David Reuben, M.D., informs his public that a clitoris 'as much as two or more inches in length when erect' is possible and that 'lesbians with this anatomical quirk are in great demand.' . . . Charlotte Wolff, M.D., notes that in lesbians it is not infrequent to find 'a habitually enlarged clitoris' that in extreme conditions resembles 'a small penis.'
>
> (Barale 1991: 242)

All three writers cited by Barale have the letters MD after their name, giving their statements the status of expert medical opinion on homosexuality.

Many well-meaning health and social care professionals are hurt and perplexed by the unwillingness of lesbian and gay clients to be open about their sexuality in interactions with care providers. Extensive research data have confirmed this unwillingness (see, for example, Stevens 1993; Sheffield Health 1996; Mugglestone 1999; Wilton 1999b), often to the frustration of those who want to offer a high standard of care to their lesbian or gay clients. This characteristic reticence becomes a little easier to understand in the context of this history of flawed, and sometimes unethical, research.

Just in case we might think that peculiar notions such as the hyper-masculine lesbian have lost their credibility with medical practitioners, the story of one British woman's experiences as recently as 1986 offers a warning that this is not necessarily the case:

> Sometimes this seemingly wilful ignorance [about lesbianism] leads to situations bordering on malpractice. A friend of mine had suffered for a long time with lumps in her breasts and other worrying symptoms. One specialist finally stumbled upon the fact of her lesbianism. He subsequently wrote to her GP saying that the problem was hormonal: as a lesbian she had 'an enlarged clitoris' and 'body hair'. In actual fact, just to put the record straight, she has neither. He wanted to prescribe hormonally: fortunately her more enlightened GP disagreed.
>
> (Hemmings 1986: 131)

This clinician, by stating in a written report that his patient has an enlarged clitoris and body hair *without even examining her,* has ignored accepted standards of clinical observation in favour of medical folklore about the manly lesbian. As Stern (1993: xii) comments, 'No wonder women are reluctant to come out [to health care staff] as lesbians – it's dangerous out there!'

The myth of the masculine lesbian, while it did not originate in medicine, continues to percolate through many aspects of clinical research and throughout health and social care arenas. In nursing, for example, it may take the form of anxiety about lesbian patients making unwanted sexual advances to female nursing staff. This fear is based on nurses' experiences of being on the receiving end of such harassment from some heterosexual male patients and on the assumption that lesbian sexuality is 'like' heterosexual male sexuality. In fact there are no cases of such behaviour on record (Webb 1985; Stevens 1993).

More technically sophisticated theories

Although the habit of measuring lesbian and gay genitalia in order to isolate their distinctively homosexual characteristics has lost favour with medical science, researchers continue to probe the bodies of lesbians and gay men in an attempt to find out what makes them prefer members of their own sex. Advances in medical technology, together with new developments in scientific thinking about the body, mean that such investigations are now carried out at a microscopic level. Nevertheless, the greater part of this recent research continues to be based on the premise that homosexuality is a malfunction of *gender,* and that it should be possible to isolate some alien element of maleness in the body of a lesbian or find a trace of femaleness in a gay man's body. The two most influential theories that have developed from this position are the hormonal and the neurological.

The hormonal theories (there is more than one) suggest that gay men are gay because they have been, at some point in their physiological development, overexposed to 'female' hormones, or underexposed to 'male' hormones. The earliest proponent of this position was Dr Clifford Wright (1892–1961), who thought that society should be tolerant of homosexuals, because homosexuality was a condition caused by a reversal in the proper proportion of 'sex hormones'. He further claimed that 'true' homosexuality could be diagnosed by hormonal assay of a blood sample, and that it could be 'cured' by hormonal treatment (Kenen 1997). None of his claims has ever been successfully proven.

Havelock Ellis first suggested that homosexuality was the result of some malfunction in the biological processes of sex development at the foetal stage. He wrote that 'a fundamental source [probably lay] in the stimulating and inhibiting play of the internal secretions' (Kenen 1997: 200). Ellis's suggestion was an informed guess; endocrinology as we know it did not then exist. By 1927 it had been discovered that so-called 'male' and 'female' hormones were present in both men and women, and this enabled Wright to suggest that it was the proportion or ratio of these hormones which was significant.

> true homosexuality is congenital in most cases and probably originates in fetal life at the time of sex determination and sex differentiation, and is markedly influenced by the endocrine glands, and, as would be expected, most of these individuals regard homosexual interest as the natural one.
>
> (Wright 1939, cited in Kenen 1997: 201)

The search for a hormonal origin for homosexuality continues right up to the present day. The most influential among contemporary researchers are an American, John Money, and a German, Gunter Dorner. Money's work grew out of his studies of andogynous infants; that is, infants born with ambivalent, imperfectly differentiated genitals. This work led him to conclude that, although there is no absolute cause-and-effect mechanism at work, adult homosexuality is most likely to be the result of a foetus receiving the 'wrong dose' of hormones *in utero*. This has led some to see maternal stress during pregnancy as leading to gay babies, although sociologists point out that, if this were the case, we could expect unusually large numbers of future lesbians and gay men to be born in the wake of major stressful events such as war or natural disaster, and that there is no evidence for this.

Dorner's work is based on experiments with rats, in which he caused male rats to adopt typically female receptive sexual postures ('lordosis') and female rats to adopt typically male mounting behaviour by exposing them to prenatal hormonal manipulation. Dorner also claimed to have demonstrated a 'positive oestrogen feedback effect' in adult gay men who had been injected with oestrogen. He concluded that his research, 'suggests that male homosexuals possess in fact, at least in part, a predominantly female-differentiated brain' (cited in Ruse 1988: 112).

It is perhaps not surprising that nobody has yet been able to replicate Dorner's findings (LeVay 1993). His work, and that of Money, has been widely criticised as suffering from 'grave methodological defects', and caused such serious concern in the scientific community that Dorner was publicly censured by his fellow sex researchers (Ruse 1988). Following a rigorous examination of the research evidence produced by Money, Dorner and their associates, Michael Ruse concluded that 'what Money's work does show is that naive links between the hormones and sexuality are almost certainly wrong' and that 'all of Dorner's work on rats and his analogies from rats to humans are conceptually confusing and should be discarded' (Ruse 1988: 116, 118). To date, studies that claim to show a causal link between homosexuality and hormones have been rejected by the scientific community as unscientific and unsound (see essays in Rosario 1997). Nevertheless, they have received substantial coverage in the press, and may still be regarded as factually accurate by many lay people, including some who are themselves lesbian or gay.

Gay and straight brains?

A second theory based on assumptions about gender comes from the work of Simon LeVay and others on brain tissue. LeVay, himself a gay man, originally specialised in optical centres of the brain and was drawn to researching homosexuality in response to the HIV/AIDS crisis in the US. He claims to have discovered, in the medial preoptic region of the hypothalamus, a small group of neurones (to be precise, one of the interstitial nuclei of the anterior hypothalamus called INAH 3), which differs in size between gay and heterosexual men. This region, LeVay claims, is smaller in both gay men and heterosexual women than it is in heterosexual men, thus suggesting some sort of link between gay men and heterosexual women.

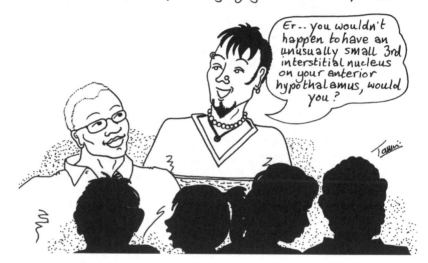

Discrete chat-up lines for today's gay man in public places --

Er -- you wouldn't happen to have an unusually small 3rd interstitial nucleus on your anterior hypothalamus, would you?

There are numerous problems with his research. First, he obtained his experimental brains from the cadavers of men who had died with AIDS, and it is well known that HIV disease can have a marked atrophying effect on brain tissue. Second, because his experimental subjects were already dead, the methods he used to determine sexual orientation were questionable. Where the clinical records showed that the probable route of acquiring HIV infection was sexual activity between men, LeVay assigned the cadaver a 'gay' identity. Where HIV infection was thought to have been acquired by a different route, he decided that they were heterosexual. He then decided to call *all* his female cadavers heterosexual, based on no firmer evidence than 'the preponderance of heterosexual women in the population' (LeVay 1993: 120).

Yet recorded routes of HIV acquisition are notoriously unreliable. Since homosexuality is so highly stigmatised, people are only too likely to lie about their sexual activities (especially where they have an investment in maintaining a heterosexual identity), and with such an extended asymptomatic period it is extremely hard to be certain of the likely route of transmission in all but the most straightforward cases (Wilton 1992). Moreover, it is clear from extensive studies that significant numbers of individual men who have casual sex with other men and/or who believe they acquired HIV through such activities, think of themselves as heterosexual (rather than gay or even bisexual), and live largely heterosexual lifestyles (Coxon 1988; Humphreys 1970; Wilton 1997a). As for the decision to assume that any dead woman is heterosexual unless proven otherwise, decades of research into the social history of lesbianism (Faraday 1981; Lesbian History Group 1989; Barrett 1990; Faderman 1991; Neild and Pearson 1992) suggest that this approach is very likely to be misleading.

In fairness, LeVay is aware of the limitations of his work. Although he glosses over the problems of his post-mortem accounting for sexual orientation, he makes clear that he does *not* believe that his work has 'proved' that homosexuality is the result of differences in brain structure. He writes (1995: 122):

> Time and again I have been described as someone who 'proved that homosexuality is genetic' . . . I did not . . . It is not possible, purely on the basis of my observations, to say whether the structural differences were present at birth, and later influenced the men to become gay or straight, or whether they arose in adult life . . .

This disclaimer does not admit to any uncertainty that there is a link of some sort between these 'structural differences' and homosexuality, nor does LeVay concede that the differences he found might have been explained in other ways. He is correct in concluding that his research *has* been interpreted as proving that homosexuality is genetic.

It is interesting that LeVay's work receives so much attention, despite serious methodological weaknesses. This suggests that the popularity of his argument is based on something other than its intrinsic validity; perhaps on its familiarity or its acceptability. Certainly there are reasons to believe that his work is perceived as credible because it is founded on the confusion between sexual orientation and biological sex which continues to underpin mainstream thinking about sexuality. In other words people believe it, despite its weaknesses, because it appears to confirm what they believe to be the case already.

If the genes fit . . .

One of the most intensive and expensive pieces of medico-scientific work ever seen is the Human Genome Project currently underway in the US. The sheer scale of the project – its annual budget is in excess of US$135 million – indicates the extent to which geneticists have succeeded in convincing politicians and the public of the value of their work. Indeed, the gene has been called the 'holy grail of the late twentieth century' (Terry 1997: 281).

Genetics has enabled medical scientists to make the kinds of optimistic claims which their forebears made on behalf of antibiotics. The promise is that unlocking the secrets of the gene will enable us to eradicate disease and disability altogether. But as well as looking for a genetic component to diseases such as breast cancer or Huntington's chorea, geneticists are also convinced that they will be able to identify genetic factors predisposing individuals to a whole range of socially problematic behaviours from violence to 'attention deficit disorder'. As Terry notes (1997: 282), 'Genetic explanations for social inequalities are extremely attractive at a time when the welfare state is in decline.'

Whatever the political issues, existing evidence for a 'gay gene' is pretty flimsy. The first team to report a genetic basis for homosexuality were psychologist Michael Bailey and psychiatrist Richard Pilger, whose work on identical twins was published in 1991. Bailey and Pilger were not geneticists. They were not even molecular biologists. Nor did they at any time use blood or tissue samples to carry out DNA testing. Their proposed 'genetic basis' for homosexuality rests on a study using a small sample of twins recruited through the gay press; roughly half the sample shared a homosexual preference.

Their method has been criticised for sampling errors, for failing to control for environmental factors and for taking at face value definitions of sexual orientation, which many social scientists would regard as naïve or anachronistic. Moreover, even taking into account the flaws in methodology, half the identical twins studied did *not* share a sexual orientation (Terry 1997). Even on its own terms, therefore, the study *disproves* a genetic basis to homosexuality just as convincingly as it proves one.

A later study, published in 1993 and carried out at the US National Cancer Institute by Dean Hamer's team, reported that it had found 'DNA markers linking male homosexuality with a region on the X chromosome [that] boys get from their mothers'. Although Hamer's research did use blood samples and microbiological technology to identify what it believed to be the significant DNA marker, it too has been criticised for many key failings. Not only did Hamer neglect to employ random samples, he also failed to carry out baseline microbiological investigations on key blood relatives such as the non-gay brothers, or even the mothers, of his gay male subjects. 'If Hamer were to have found the marker in a significant number of heterosexual brothers or mothers', comments Jennifer Terry, 'his findings of a genetic influence for homosexuality would have been seriously weakened' (1997: 286). Given this lack of scientific rigour, it is perhaps not surprising that other scientists have not been able to reproduce Hamer's findings (Allen 1997; Pillard 1997).

Implications for health and well-being

This brief history of scientific thinking about sexuality demonstrates the extent to which socio-cultural factors have influenced not only the social organisation of sexual behaviour, but also attempts on the part of scientists to find a logical explanation for homosexuality. It would be surprising if this were not the case – science does not and cannot exist in a vacuum. In order to understand some of the implications of this situation, we also have to think about power.

Social scientists and social historians regard both religion and science as – among other things – important instruments of social control. As such, they tend to have a particularly powerful impact on the lives of women and other marginalised groups. Since Foucault, historians have recognised that sexuality has been a key element in this process of social control.

Social historians point out, for example, that women fighting for equality with men have often been called lesbians (Millett 1970; Faderman 1981; Jeffreys 1985), or have been accused of wanting to *be* men. Psychology and psychiatry have been especially guilty of these strategies:

> analyst Karl Abraham . . . first interpreted the feminist movement . . . as the expression of a 'masculinity complex' in neurotic women. In the famous paper he gave at the postwar psychoanalytical congress . . . 'Manifestations of the Female Castration Complex', Abraham described feminists as women who sublimated their wish to be men by 'following masculine pursuits of an intellectual and professional nature'.
>
> (Showalter 1987: 199)

The inequalities that divide Western societies – race, socio-economic class, gender, etc. – were explained in Darwinian terms of natural selection and heredity by the eugenics movement in the early part of the twentieth century, and concerned commentators perceive that genetic arguments are being employed in a disturbingly similar way today:

> The power of the gene as a cultural icon reflects the appeal of scientific explanations that reinforce and legitimate existing social categories . . . Molecular genetics, behavioural genetics, neurobiology, and sociobiology have provided a language through which group differences that are culturally desirable [to the majority] can be interpreted as biologically determined.
>
> (Nelkin and Lindee 1995: 388)

Medicalisation and practice

It is clear from the literature that many of the difficulties facing lesbian and gay service users stem from the medicalisation of homosexuality (see, for example, Kitzinger 1987; Jessop and Thorogood 1989; Whatley 1992; Waldby 1996; Farquhar 1999). This presents particular problems for those whose professional identity and practice may be rooted in medicine.

Those initially responsible for the medicalisation of homosexuality aimed to improve the lives of homosexual people by demonstrating that they were neither criminal nor immoral but simply the innocent victims of biological malfunction. But, as we have seen, the disease model of same-sex desire, although it had some liberatory potential (Plummer 1981; Weeks 1990), also had some disastrous consequences. It set in motion a research programme focused on questions of aetiology, symptomatology and (inevitably) cure. It also contributed to the discourse of homosexuality-as-sickness, which continues to undermine attempts to provide unbiased care (Farquhar 1999). It is, for example, difficult to imagine how unbiased care may be given by those who agree with the British doctor who claimed that homosexuality is 'biologically destructive' (Rayner 1994).

The search for a 'cure'

It must also be acknowledged that the disease model of homosexuality has been put to catastrophic uses in the not too distant past. Of these, by far the worst occurred when homosexual inmates of the death camps were used as living experimental subjects by Nazi doctors eager to discover a means of curing homosexuality (Fernbach 1980; Heger 1980; Grau 1995; Miller 1995; Proctor 1995).

Since the Second World War, clinicians of many specialisms have tried, without success, to develop such a cure. They experimented with a range of 'treatments' including chemical castration, electro-convulsive therapy, surgical removal of the hypothalamus, pre-frontal lobotomy, hormone injections and clitoridectomy (Haldemann 1991; Silverstein 1991). Lesbians have been subjected to therapeutic regimes that include forcible heterosexual intercourse, and various forms of aversion therapy have been employed, using nausea-inducing drugs and even (in one notorious case) inflicting burns to the hands of patients (Ruse 1988; Silverstein 1991; Gibson 1997).

Such abuses are now largely discredited. However, young lesbians and gay men are still sometimes subjected to psychiatric treatment or detained in psychiatric institutions at the insistence of parents or guardians, anxious that their homosexuality be rectified (Miller 1995; McFarlane 1998; Institute of Medicine 1999). Rock journalist Phil Sutcliffe (1999: 78) recounts the case of Lou Reed:

> When he was 17, Reed's parents sent him to a psychiatrist to be 'cured' of homosexuality. The shrink said electric shock treatment should do the trick. Twenty-four brain frazzlings later, Reed emerged traumatised, but still gay.

Attempts to cure homosexuality have largely been abandoned. The disease model of homosexuality has itself lost credibility, with the notable exception of the evangelical 'ex-gay' movement, whose practitioners continue to draw on pathological concepts of homosexuality derived from biomedicine (Haldeman 1991; Thompson 1994; Green *et al.* 1996).

However, medical researchers continue to carry out experiments designed to prove the existence of physiological differences between homosexuals and heterosexuals (Hamer and Copeland 1994; LeVay 1996). *The Sunday Times*, for example, recently reported that: 'British scientists . . . have found that gay men's fingerprints are more similar to women's than they are to heterosexual men's' (Brennan 1998: 7). This project was funded by the Wellcome Trust, a medical research charity. In a similar vein, another group of researchers claim to have found that the relative length of lesbians' fingers is 'masculine' (Gardiner 2000).

Of course, earlier claims to have located physiological markers of this kind have foundered on the rocks of poor research design and, to date, none has been replicated (Ruse 1988; Rosario 1997). Given that a growing body of social scientific research data points to a fluid, shifting and flexible account of sexual preference (Stein 1993; Whisman 1996; Farquhar 1999), it seems increasingly unlikely that physiological differences, such as the 'pink thumbprint' (Brennan 1998) will hold up to rigorous scrutiny. There remains an interesting ethical debate to be had concerning the rationale for continuing to fund biomedical research of this kind.

Conclusion: a political paradox

What biomedical theories of sexual orientation have in common is *essentialism*, a belief that sexuality is an essential, or innate, component of individual biological makeup. From the historical perspective of a decades-old fight for the civil and human rights of lesbians and gay men, the impact of the essentialist approach has been paradoxical. It can be used both to support change and to prevent it.

It was, after all, the essentialist theories of the early sexologists that lent sufficient coherence to the idea of the homosexual for individuals to start building both a sense of personal identity and a supportive community around that idea. For many lesbians and gay men today, that sense of identity and the existence of that community offer a sense of safety and sanctuary which is desperately needed in a hostile world. As Plummer (1981: 29) concludes, 'with all these categorizations comes the paradox: they control, restrict and inhibit whilst simultaneously providing comfort, security and assuredness.'

Belief that homosexuality is innate – we are born this way – or that it is unchangeably fixed by a very young age, has underpinned a key strand of the demand for civil and human rights. The argument has been that it is unjust and inhumane to exclude and persecute people for something over which they have no control. Moreover the belief that homosexuality is fixed and innate frees the community from the attentions of many of its enemies. A biological characteristic cannot be immoral or sinful, which makes religious fundamentalist attacks on gay people meaningless. If sexual orientation is innate or is fixed by the age of three or five years, then it makes no sense to prohibit lesbians and gay men from being teachers, youth workers, social workers or parents. If sexual orientation cannot be changed, this offers an escape route from those psychiatrists who still insist that homosexuality is a personality disorder which may be cured.

This is especially important in the US, where right-wing fundamentalism is extraordinarily powerful and determined to eradicate homosexuality:

> Fundamentalist propaganda incites . . . violence. Anita Bryant, leader of the 'Save Our Children' campaign, announced that 'God puts homosexuals in the same category as murderers.' A mass mailing from Reverend Jerry Falwell . . . called on readers to 'Stop the Gays *dead* in their perverted tracks.' Dean Wycoff of the Santa Clara branch of the Moral Majority stated on television that he believed that 'homosexuality should be included with murder and other capital crimes so that the government that sits upon this land would be doing the executing.' Episodes of [anti-gay] violence jumped following this.
>
> (Greenberg 1988: 467. Emphasis in Falwell original)

It is not surprising that some sections of the gay community are keen to adopt an approach which seems to offer a legitimate defence against such dangerous adversaries. Indeed, essentialist arguments have been an important factor in decriminalisation, and in campaigns to equalise the age of consent.

Others, however, point to weaknesses in the traditional dependence on essentialism. Racism, sexism, ageism and the social exclusion of disabled people are all based on physical characteristics over which individuals have no control, and there is no reason to imagine that homosexuality should be an exception to this rule.

In the age of the gene, any claim that homosexuality is biological begins to look frightening. According to Allen, it is not only lesbians and gay men who are alarmed by the prospect of genetic testing for a 'gay gene':

> Even . . . neurobiologist Roger Gorski, who believes strongly that male and female brains are hardwired for gender roles, has remarked that '[t]here is something reductive and scary about a situation in which you *might* be able to ask a mother whether she wants testosterone treatment to avoid having a homsexual son.'
>
> (Allen 1997: 242)

Clearly, even those working within the paradigm of biological essentialism are disturbed by the potential applications of such research. This suggests that those with most to lose – in this case the lesbian and gay community – need to think extremely carefully about the long-term consequences of supporting essentialist claims.

A different approach altogether is taken by a more radical strand of activists. They suggest that, rather than merely aiming for tolerance of lesbian, gay and bisexual people, the entire social organisation of sexuality needs to be rethought. This, they argue, should be done in such a way that all individuals are able to make real choices – including the choice to be straight or gay. For example, some lesbian feminists argue that it may be politically important for women to devote their emotional and sexual energies to other women, rather than to men (Hoagland 1988). This approach has little time for essentialist theories.

Whatever the political implications, debates about the origin of sexual orientation will doubtless continue. In the professional context of health and social care what matters is not so much deciding which theory is 'right', but applying a critical perspective to scientific research in this field. It is especially important to understand the broader social implications of medical models of homosexuality, as well as their potential consequences for the emotional health and well-being of service users.

---

exercise

Read the following passage taken from Simon LeVay's (1996) book, *Queer Science: The Uses and Abuses of Research into Homosexuality.*

Hall and Kimura tested the accuracy of heterosexual men and women in throwing a ball to a target. They confirmed the basic sex difference in the task (the heterosexual men were significantly more accurate than the heterosexual women), but they also found that the gay men were significantly less accurate than the straight men; in fact, they were about as bad as the heterosexual women. Conversely, the lesbians did *better* than heterosexual women, although the difference did not quite reach statistical significance.

What assumptions underpinned the research? What questions need to be asked about matters such as sampling, sample size, definitions of sexual orientation used or nature of task set? The researchers concluded that their findings support a biological basis for homosexuality. What other explanations can you think of for the differences in performance they describe? How might you test other explanations experimentally?

Further reading

Hamer, D. and Copeland, P. (1994) *The Science of Desire: The Search for the Gay Gene and the Biology of Behaviour*. New York: Simon & Schuster.

LeVay, S. (1993) *The Sexual Brain*. Cambridge, MA: Massachusetts Institute of Technology Press.

Mort, F. (1987) *Dangerous Sexualities: Medico-Moral Politics in England since 1830*. London: Routledge & Kegan Paul.

Rosario, V. (ed.) (1997) *Science and Homosexualities*. London: Routledge.

Ruse, M. (1988) *Homosexuality: A Philosophical Inquiry*. Oxford: Basil Blackwell.

Terry, J. and Urla, J. (eds) (1995) *Deviant Bodies: Critical Perspectives on Difference in Science and Popular Culture*. Indianapolis, IN: Indiana University Press.

5 social theories: development and debates

Introduction

Just as social explanations of ill health depart from a purely biomedical model, so sociological theories of sexuality are very different from those which underpin the kinds of research discussed in the previous chapter. Beginning with an explanation of the development and nature of the sociology of sexuality, this chapter goes on to discuss its links with social movements such as feminism and gay liberation. It continues with a brief overview of the consequences of newer, social constructionist, models of sexuality for the lesbian and gay community, for their human rights, their well-being and their sense of identity. In conclusion, it outlines some implications for health and social care practice.

The nature of sociological questions

The theories discussed in the previous chapter may all be loosely termed *essentialist*, insofar as they all assume the existence of a homosexual (and a heterosexual) *essence* of some kind. Whether their concerns are with hormones, neurophysiology or genital structure, they all share a belief that there is fundamental *difference in kind* between heterosexuals and homosexuals, that sexual orientation is an essential characteristic of individuals, and as such it makes sense to search for its trace, if not its cause, in the human body.

Essentialist theories of sexuality tend to be closely associated with medicalisation, since the fundamental premise – that there is a homosexual 'condition' of some kind (there is seldom much concern with the heterosexual equivalent) – leads fairly directly into a concern for causes, distinguishing features, consequences and strategies for prevention. This neatly parallels the clinical model of disease; aetiology, symptomatology, clinical prognosis and questions of prevention and cure.

It is important to state at the outset that, although essentialist and social explanations are *competing paradigms*, they are not mutually exclusive. Most social scientists accept that biology is likely to play some part, however small, in shaping sexuality. For example, Greenberg concludes (1988: 487) that 'The years some homosexuals spend trying without success to conform to conventional expectations regarding gender and sexual orientation tell against the more extreme claims of sexual plasticity.' Similarly, no geneticist or neurologist has yet claimed that biology *determines* sexual orientation. On the contrary, they have generally been scrupulous in insisting that biology is only one factor involved in the genesis of a sexual orientation (LeVay 1996).

Questions of scale

The key distinction between the two paradigms is one of levels of analysis. Essentialist theories have tended to emerge within disciplines whose primary focus is relatively small-scale. Endocrinology – the scientific study of hormones – confines itself to the level of the individual body, as do the other biomedical sciences such as neurology. This makes them extremely useful when trying to discover, for example, what effect a lesion on the thyroid gland might have. However, they are less useful tools for investigating entire societies. You would not expect a neurologist, for example, to explain capitalism as a function of neural activity. As we have seen, human sexuality is enmeshed in complex social, cultural and political structures, all of which are continually shifting. In this context, trying to understand sexuality by looking at chromosomes or brain structure is analogous to trying to understand Verdi's operas by carrying out a biopsy of Placido Domingo's vocal chords.

Social scientists have accumulated a varied body of data about sexuality, much of which calls into question the certainties of essentialist theories. For example, detailed studies of non-industrial cultures have shown that categories such as heterosexuality and homosexuality are not human universals (Caplan 1987; Ramet 1996).

Different meanings for same-sex activity have evolved in different cultures. For some, more or less ritualised same-sex acts are a necessary part of the journey from childhood to adulthood. Some societies make no connection between same-sex activity and gender-role non-compliance, whereas others clearly do. Some, as we have seen, have even created appropriate social roles and cultural rituals for such individuals. Such findings seriously weaken claims, whether within biomedicine or psychology, that some universal process is at work to make individuals homosexual or heterosexual (Ruse 1988).

Once it is recognised that sexual behaviours and customs vary from place to place and are liable to change over time, essentialist theories lose much of their coherence. For example, the Sambia people of New Guinea believe that no boy can become an adult man and marry unless he has imbibed an adequate quantity of semen by fellating older men during puberty rituals (Pillard 1997). It seems fairly pointless to think in terms of tracking down a 'gay gene' or structural anomaly in brain tissue that predisposes the Sambia to behave in this way, since trying to squeeze this particular form of same-sex activity into a Western concept of homosexuality (or, indeed, of paedophilia) just does not work. If we are to understand how such historical and cultural elements shape sexuality, we require a much more large-scale focus than essentialist theories have to offer, and this is where sociology comes in.

A history of the sociology of sexuality

Early sociological studies of homosexuality were constrained by its criminal status. Where certain sexual behaviours are illegal there are consequences for the behaviour of *all* individuals in that society at that time. It may with some certainty be predicted that such activities will be secretive, strongly bound up with fear, guilt and the potential for blackmail, and that fewer people will have the confidence, courage or recklessness to carry them out, whatever their desires. If homosexual acts are crimes, those who engage in them are thereby criminalised. The familiar elements of a gay subculture become, under such circumstances, part of a *criminal* subculture. The sociologist exploring homosexuality under such conditions is engaged perforce in studying a secretive underworld. As Johnston wrote (1973: 58), in America in the 1950s, 'there was no lesbian [or gay] identity except a criminal one', and the same was true in Britain and many other European countries.

The human zoo

The early study of lesbian and gay people was, therefore, guided by the same principles used when studying drug addicts, prostitutes and other criminals, and relied on the same broad theoretical perspective, sometimes termed the sociology of deviance. The homosexual underworld was like a fish-bowl, with sociologists, psychologists and others peering in from the outside, interpreting what they saw from the dominant heterosexual perspective.

Objectivity was a difficult achievement against a background of very negative attitudes. In 1970, a national survey was conducted in the US for the Institute for Sex Research. Forty-nine per cent of the respondents agreed with the statement 'homosexuality is a social corruption which can cause the downfall of a civilisation' (cited in Greenberg 1988: 457). It would be very challenging to develop an unbiased research practice against such a negative social background.

Labelling theory

The most enduring approach that developed from work carried out within the sociology of deviance was *labelling theory*. This approach was employed to examine many forms of social deviance and eventually became useful in constructing social models of mental illness and disability (Plummer 1981; Hevey 1992). Labelling theory is complex, but its two key premises, as summarised by Abercrombie *et al.* (1994: 132) are:

> that deviant behaviour is to be seen not simply as the violation of a norm, but as any behaviour which is successfully defined or labelled as deviant. The deviance does not inhere in the act itself, but in the response of others to that act. The second proposition claims that labelling produces or amplifies deviance. The deviant's response to societal reaction leads to secondary deviation by which the deviant comes to accept a self-image or self-definition as someone who is permanently locked within a deviant role.

In other words, if one man sucks another's penis, the act is not enough *in itself* to cause him to think of himself as 'homosexual'. If he is a Sambia adolescent, he will simply think of himself as an adult man, since that is how the act, and persons performing it, are 'labelled' in Sambia culture. If he is a British adolescent, however, the consequences of the act depend on other cultural variables. He may be aware of 'expert' opinion that it is normal for adolescents to go through an experimental homosexual 'phase', in which case his sense of his own normality may be reinforced. On the other hand, if his experience becomes labelled 'homosexual', whether by his peers, parents or adult authority figures or by comparison with media and press images, he may begin to think of *himself* as homosexual, and then to act out his perceptions of a homosexual 'role'.

This stage of acting out is referred to in the sociological literature as 'secondary deviance'. Labelling is very significant for the future identity and life choices of the individual, since it strongly influences the extent to which they adopt, or resist adopting, a 'deviant career'. In the case of homosexuality, the individual who is labelled 'gay' is clearly more likely to seek out a gay community than one who accepts the 'experimental phase' label for their experiences. Of course, the labelling responses of others are not the *only* influence at work. A whole range of other factors – psychological, social, cultural or spiritual – are likely to be involved.

Labelling theory grew out of a broader theoretical school within sociology, known as *symbolic interactionism*. This started with the work of George Herbert Mead, who conceived of society as an interactive exchange of gestures (speech, dress, body language, written language) involving the use of meaningful symbols. Its area of study is the relationship between the self and society, and both 'self' and 'society' are understood to be *produced* by symbolic interactions (i.e. meaningful communication) between social actors (individuals, groups and institutions). In terms of sexuality, symbolic interactionism offers insights into the origin of ideas such as 'lesbian' or 'heterosexual', and what their consequences are for the ways in which individuals and social groups make sense of themselves and the wider world.

Paradigm shift: knowledge and politics

Social scientific 'knowledge' is closely interwoven with processes of social change, and this is perhaps especially true with regard to sexuality. After all, the study of homosexuality requires the existence of individuals who accept this label for themselves and who are accessible to researchers, something that can only happen in certain places and at certain times. This is true, to a certain extent, of essentialist models too. As Greenberg points out, even the medical model must be recognised as a product of *interactions* between the medical community and the embryonic gay community:

> physicians did not invent the notion of an essential homosexuality. It was a product of the urban male-homosexual networks and sub-cultures that had developed in European cities well before the late

nineteenth century. The participants in those subculture contributed actively to the development of what eventually came to be called a 'medical' conception of homosexuality.

(Greenberg 1988: 486)

Wider social and cultural changes, pre-eminently urbanisation, industrial-isation and the growth of capitalism, were influential in enabling men and (to a lesser degree) women with same-sex desires to gather together for the first time, and to begin organising their *identities* around those desires (Katz 1983; Donoghue 1993; Chauncey 1994; McCormick 1997). As Greenberg understands it, the medical model grew out of the meanings that became attached to same-sex desire in the context of this fragile new subculture, both by outsiders looking in and by the participants themselves. Similarly, the great shift in thinking about sexuality which started in the late 1960s could not have taken place without massive changes in the lesbian and gay community; on the other hand, when those shifts in thinking did take place they themselves contributed to the growing trans-formations of the community under study.

The 1960s were a time of great social upheaval and of rapid changes in belief systems and social organisation throughout the West. This time of change was marked in the lesbian and gay community by a move away from assimilationist politics towards a greater militancy. Up to this point, political activism had been directed towards decriminalisation, and gay campaigners sought acceptance from wider heterosexual society. Organisa-tions such as (in the UK) the Homosexual Law Reform Society and the Campaign for Homosexual Equality or (in the US) the Mattachine Society and the early lesbian organisation, the Daughters of Bilitis, tried to present a non-threatening image of homosexuals as exemplary citizens who only wished for understanding and tolerance. At this time, the theories of the early sexologists were extremely popular among lesbians and gay men, since they explained homosexuality as something which was outside the voluntary control of the individual and therefore not anyone's fault (Weeks 1990).

The 1960s and Stonewall

All this changed with the new social movements of the 1960s, in particular the rise of feminism and Black Power. Feminists set out to demonstrate that there was nothing natural about gender roles or men's power over women. At the same time, Black activists were discarding the old, apologetic 'Uncle Tom' image in favour of the declaration that 'Black is Beautiful'. The implication of these new kinds of activism was that the 'differences' which had traditionally been used to justify the oppression of women and Blacks were social and political rather than biological, a realisation that was not lost on the embryonic gay movement (Altman 1993).

In terms of sexuality, the historical moment that marks the point of transition is often taken to be the Stonewall uprising. The Stonewall Inn was a gay bar in Greenwich Village, New York, accustomed to random raids and harrassment by the police. On 27 June 1969, there was another routine raid. This time, however, the patrons of the Stonewall fought back. Fed up with victimisation, New York's gay community rioted for four days. Although the news media of the time suppressed the story, shockwaves from Stonewall spread slowly across the gay community in the English-speaking world (Thompson 1994). It signalled a mood of defiance, which was to underpin the foundations of a new lesbian and gay politics, to the extent that social historians speak of the 'pre-Stonewall era' and 'post-Stonewall era' as recognisably distinct. Just as 'Black is Beautiful' had served as a rallying cry for the Black Power movement, so 'Gay is Good' became the slogan of the post-Stonewall gay movement, as the newly radical Gay Liberation Front came into being.

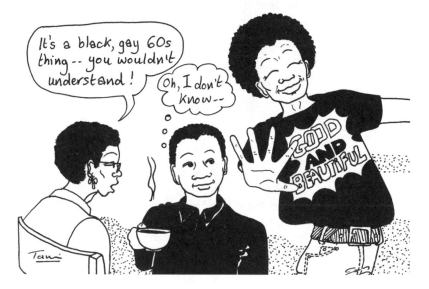

The startling shift in this new approach to civil rights was the claim that there was positive value in being different, and this led to shifts in the whole notion of what 'difference' meant. Although very little of what sprang directly from the new social movements could be thought of as social science, it is nevertheless possible to spot the origins of much of today's sophisticated social scientific theories in some of the political writings of the time.

For example, in 1970 a breakaway feminist group called the Radicalesbians published a statement, *The Woman Identified Woman* (reprinted in Lucia-Hoagland and Penelope 1988) in which they wrote:

> It should first be understood that lesbianism, like male homosexuality, is a category of behaviour possible only in a sexist society characterized by rigid sex roles and dominated by male supremacy . . . Homosexuality is a by-product of a particular way of setting up roles (or approved patterns of behaviour) on the basis of sex . . . In a society in which

men do not oppress women, and sexual expression is allowed to follow feelings, the categories of homosexuality and heterosexuality would disappear.

(Lucia-Hoagland and Penelope 1988: 17–18)

This is not an academic paper, but it contains the seeds of a key shift in thinking about sexuality. The debates taking place in the lesbian and gay community at the time became the raw material of more formal social constructionist theories, and of a sociology of homosexuality that focused on oppression. As British sociologist Ken Plummer (1981: 26) comments:

We should be clear then that it was only once the sociologists got near to the gay movement and heard the debates (and in many cases – myself included – 'gays' and 'sociologists' became synomymous) that they were able to pose the additional questions of 'gay oppression'. It is interesting to ponder whether sociologists would have asked such questions had a gay movement never occurred.

The paradigm shift, as Plummer indicates, was at least partly a consequence of the gradually increasing confidence of professional sociologists who were themselves gay or lesbian, and who, following the partial decrimin-alisation of homosexuality and the assertiveness of the post-Stonewall community, were able to be more open about their own sexuality. No longer was the lesbian and gay community a fish-bowl being studied by outsiders, the sociologists were swimming right alongside. Traditional questions along the lines of 'Gosh, those goldfish are swimming in circles, I wonder why?', were replaced by others: 'What effect does it have on the swimming behaviour of a goldfish if you put it in a little bowl?' and 'If *they* think they have the right to put us in this bowl in the first place, what does that say about *them*?' In other words, it was no longer possible simply to frame questions with homosexuality as the problem; the very process of categorising sexualities came under scrutiny.

Social constructionism

Social constructionists are less interested in studying social events than in identifying the social and cultural mechanisms that enable sense to be made of such events, and in assessing the consequences of the meanings which are so created. Their four main assumptions (from Gergen 1985) are:

1 The way we go about studying the world is determined by available concepts, categories and methods.
2 The concepts and categories we use vary considerably in their meaning and connotations over time and across cultures.
3 The popularity or persistence of any category, concept or method depends more on its *usefulness* (especially its *political* usefulness) than on its intrinsic validity.

4 Descriptions and explanations of the world are themselves social actions, and have social consequences.

The first two assumptions are relatively straightforward. For example, it was obviously not possible for physicians in the fifteenth century to study the immunological significance of white blood cells, since they lacked the concepts of an immune response or of cells, and did not have access to microscopes and other necessary apparatus. Similarly, our ability to examine certain social interactions is restricted by available concepts of gender.

It is also quite easy to accept the second assumption, since our daily lives teach us that concepts and categories vary in their meaning and connotations. For example, the fact that you can buy aspirin in Boots does not mean that their staff are 'drug dealers'. It is the third and fourth assumptions that give social constructionism its theoretical edge over earlier perspectives. They are also more difficult to accept at face value.

To assert that a category (such as 'homosexuality'), a concept (such as 'family'), or a method (such as psychiatric classification) persists because of its political usefulness rather than because it is 'accurate' or 'right' has two important implications. The first is that all of them must involve *power* and, to a greater or lesser degree, vested interests. This may be an uncomfortable realisation, since it casts doubt over such notions as rationality or scientific objectivity.

The second implication is that 'truth' is not something 'real', which exists and needs to be found. Rather, it is *produced*. What you 'discover' is, to a large extent, the end product of the means you have used to look for it – and these are determined by their political usefulness. For example, if you use the tools of genetics to look for criminality, you will not be able to find out anything about the impact of social deprivation. It does not take much political sophistication to work out that this may have a direct bearing on funding!

The fourth assumption of social constructionism, that descriptions and explanations of the world are social actions with social consequences, has enormous implications. It means that labelling anything is never a neutral, value-free act, because the very act of labelling produces effects. For example, the decision to label alcoholism a disease – rather than a moral failing – transformed the way in which alcoholics are treated and their perceptions of themselves and generated a multi-million dollar clinical industry.

The homosexual role

Social constructionism is a very powerful set of tools for *deconstructing* social interactions. How did it develop in the context of the sociology of sexuality? *The Homosexual Role*, an essay first published in 1968 by British sociologist Mary McIntosh, is generally credited as the catalyst (Altman 1993). Of course, this seminal essay did not emerge in a vacuum. It was preceded by some important earlier work in the US, which had established two radical ideas. Sociologists Leznoff and Westley had begun to shift the emphasis from homosexuality-as-pathology to the social relations that structured the lived experience of their gay contemporaries. They commented that 'The subjection of homosexuals to legal punishment and social condemnation has produced a complex structure of concealed social relations which merit sociological investigation' (Leznoff and Westley 1967: 185). Social psychologist Evelyn Hooker was carrying out a battery of established psychological tests on lesbian and gay subjects, which led her to conclude, not simply that they were psychologically 'normal' and healthy, but that the supposed clinical entity 'homosexuality' did not exist in the first place (Plummer 1981).

Taken together, these insights from different disciplines laid the foundation for McIntosh's suggestion that homosexuality was a social role *produced by* the 'complex structure of concealed social relations', which Leznoff and Westley had proposed studying. Moreover, as McIntosh herself pointed out, Alfred Kinsey's pioneering work had led him to reject the homo/hetero sexual divide as long ago as 1948. Kinsey *et al.* (1948: 637) explicitly dismissed the idea that 'every individual is innately – inherently – either heterosexual or homosexual', proposing instead the now familiar 'Kinsey scale', which allowed individuals to position themselves anywhere on a continuum between exclusive heterosexuality at one pole and exclusive homosexuality at the other. Most of us, according to Kinsey, fall somewhere in between. The notion of a scale was quite quickly absorbed into popular thinking, perhaps especially amongst gay men (who still sometimes refer to themselves as 'a Kinsey 8' or 'a Kinsey 6'), but it did not result in a general rejection of the belief that homosexuals and heterosexuals are distinct groups of people.

The continuation of such beliefs, despite a mass of empirical evidence contradicting them and mounting evidence of serious methodological flaws in the empirical research that claimed to support them, was what interested McIntosh and her colleagues. Distinguishing between homosexual behaviour and what she termed the homosexual *role* enabled McIntosh to propose 'that the homosexual should be seen as playing a social role rather than as having a condition' (1968: 33). Moreover, she began to identify this social role as one which had a socio-political *function*:

> The vantage point of comparative sociology enables us to see that the conception of homosexuality as a condition is, in itself, a possible object of study. This conception and the behaviour it supports operate as a form of social control in a society in which homosexuality is condemned.
>
> (McIntosh 1968: 31)

From this perspective, as outlined by McIntosh, it becomes possible to investigate how sexual desire and activity between members of the same biological sex came to be *called* 'homosexuality', how the idea of homosexuality is maintained, which groups have a vested interest in maintaining it and which in challenging it and what the implications are for the categories of people *created* by this idea (namely, homosexuals, hetero-sexuals and the residual category of bisexuals) and for the social organisa-tion of sexuality. In other words, once scientists such as Kinsey, Hooker and others had established that homosexuality is not 'real', in the sense of a discrete set of personal characteristics detectable through empirical observation, McIntosh was able to see it as a *social construct*, an idea constructed by social interactions of all kinds.

Foucault

The most radical social-constructionist account of sexuality came from Michel Foucault, a French historian of ideas, who pin-pointed the invention of the homosexual in the nineteenth century. In what has become one of the most-quoted passages ever written about sexuality, he explains:

> The nineteenth-century homosexual became a personage, a past, a case history and a childhood, in addition to being a type of life, a life form, and a morphology, with an indiscreet anatomy and possibly a mysterious physiology . . . Homosexuality appeared as one of the forms of sexuality when it was transposed from the practice of sodomy onto a kind of interior androgyny, a hermaphrodism of the soul. The sodomite had been a temporary aberration; the homosexual was now a species.
>
> (Foucault 1976: 43)

Although historians have subsequently modified Foucault's account, his analysis of the ways in which different forms of socio-political *power* may be observed at work in the social organisation of sexuality has been widely accepted by social scientists. What was remarkable about Foucault's work was that he moved a crucial step beyond seeing sex as a basic human instinct, repressed by those in power. Foucault proposed that it is in the interests of certain groups to promulgate the idea that sex is a basic instinct in the first place. This idea itself must therefore be recognised as a social construct. The significant shift that Foucault initiated was from seeing sex as *exploited* in the interests of powerful groups to seeing sex as *produced* through discourse by the operations of power. This meant that different discourses, exemplified in everything from pop songs to medical textbooks, could contribute to a wider *social construction* of sexuality. This is the central concept of social constructionism.

Implications for human rights

The implications of this social constructionist model of sexuality are dra-matic. Recognising that explanations of the world are social acts with social consequences offers a critical new perspective on essentialist accounts. Specifically, it enables different theoretical perspectives to be recognised as political (in the broadest sense of the word).

Sometimes the political implications are very stark, as Garland Allen suggests in his paper on the history of genetic determinism (Allen 1997). In a telling demonstration of how important it can be to set scientific research in its historical and political context, Allen reminds us that the US sheltered many Nazi scientists, granting them immunity from prosecution for war crimes, and that this collaboration eventually produced the genetics research establishment in the US today.

Allen suggests that this history may help to explain why genetic explanations of behaviour remain so influential in the US, despite the fact that 'None of [their] claims have ever withstood close scrutiny' (Allen 1997: 243). He continues with a rigorous examination of genetic theories of homosexuality, concluding that:

> Despite difference in subject matter or historical period, theories of genetic determinism have shared a variety of methodological pitfalls that recur time and time again, despite clear and overt criticism. It is as if these theories have had no history . . . [furthermore] they have more often led to restricting human opportunity . . . than to enhancing it, more often to reinforcing cultural prejudices than to overriding them.

Allen is not, of course, suggesting that genetics is a fascist science, merely that its current power and credibility owes as much to politics as to its usefulness as a tool for explaining human behaviours.

The rigorous critical analysis of continuing attempts to categorise people according to their desires has effectively undermined the logic of essentialism. However, biomedical scientists and social scientists tend to inhabit very segregated professional and disciplinary worlds, and what appears as a resounding defeat of biomedical explanations in social constructionist circles does not appear to have had much impact on the research agendas of biomedicine.

The political implications have been important in other ways. As Plummer suggests, once essentialist categories are recognised as sociopolitical, the exclusion of lesbians and gay men is no longer defensible in a democracy. He writes:

> Certainly there is considerable political intent behind the making of such categorisations – to order, control and segregate in the name of benevolence . . . Certainly too these categories have rendered – in the main – whole groups of people devalued, dishonourable or dangerous, and have frequently justified monstrous human atrocities and the denial of human rights.
>
> (Plummer 1981: 53)

However, just as essentialists and constructionists inhabit different worlds, so too do academics and the people they write about. Whilst many lesbian and gay academics welcome the demolition of essentialist accounts, it is important to remember that essentialism developed in close association with the developing gay subculture. We might therefore expect that anti-essentialist accounts would meet with some hostility in the lesbian and gay community, and this has indeed been the case.

Problems and debates in the community

It is not surprising that social constructionism has been the subject of heated debate in the lesbian and gay community. After all, it has proved controversial in academic circles (Stein 1990) and has not been widely discussed in the press or media. The main exception to this has been the feminist assertion that gender is a social construct, which led to widespread and continuing concern amongst educationalists, parents and politicians, about the ways in which boys and girls are socialised into narrow and restrictive roles in adult life (see, for example, Oakley 1972; Whyte *et al.* 1985; Arnot and Weiner 1987; Weiner and Arnot 1987).

Essentialism and gay politics

Many people react to social constructionism with suspicion and unease. After all, as Vance reminds us (1981: 13), the rug under our feet is being shaken:

> Social constructionist theory in the field of sexuality proposed an extremely outrageous idea. It suggested that one of the last remaining outposts of the 'natural' in our thinking was fluid and changeable, the product of human action and history rather than the invariant result of the body, biology, or an innate sex drive.

The implications of constructionism are pretty uncomfortable. If our sexuality is *not*, after all, an irresistible drive, we are required to take a much greater degree of responsibility for our sexual behaviour. Moreover, as Greenberg points out, if you have spent your life trying to live according to familiar 'rules' of gender and sexuality then it may be hurtful to your self-esteem and sense of values, as well as intellectually disruptive, to see those rules overthrown. This, he suggests, is what lies behind the American finding that the most homophobic individuals are those with the most conservative lifestyles:

> For many Americans, adherence to conventional values and standards was a major component of their claim to respectability. The challenge to conventionality was therefore an implicit – and sometimes explicit – attack on this claim . . . The activist who chanted 'gay is twice as good as straight' denied straights their claim to being morally worthy *for not being homosexual*. People with other sources of self-regard could perhaps shrug off this denial. But to others, such as those whose material success has been limited, moral respectabilty has been psychologically important.
>
> (Greenberg 1988: 473. My italics)

Shifting sands

For those who define themselves as lesbian or gay, social constructionism seemed to pose a still more annihilating threat. There is a crucial
psychological element in coming to terms with the outsider status of a
lesbian or gay identity. As Terry puts it (1997: 273): 'We, as deviant
subjects, have to account for ourselves as anomalies. We are compelled to
ask certain *questions of the self*, beyond the generic question of Who am I?'
Forging an identity as a lesbian or gay man, and establishing some kind
of relationship with the lesbian and gay community – even if the relationship consists in rejecting that community and its norms – is a necessary
psychological strategy in such circumstances. Having gone through such
psychological upheaval, it is of little comfort to be told that your hard-
won identity is somehow fictitious.

Politically, too, many lesbians and gay men have felt that deconstructing
a homosexual identity undermines the very basis of arguments for equality.
If there is no such thing as a 'real' lesbian or gay man, how is it possible
to argue that such people have been deprived of their human and civil
rights (Fuss 1989; Whisman 1996)?

Gender differences

There are also important gender differences that need to be taken into
account. Women and men do not generally experience their sexuality in
the same way (Schwartz and Rutter 1998). Lesbians and gay men do not
necessarily have anything in common other than the label 'homosexual'.
Enough research has now been done to enable us to say that such differences seem to run very deep. For example, whilst it is relatively common
for lesbians to experience their sexuality as a matter of personal choice,
such accounts are rare amongst gay men, who are far more likely to feel
that their orientation was fixed at a very early age (Whisman 1996;
Wilton 1999b). As Terry found (1997: 281), 'Some gay men's narratives
of "having always felt this way" are very powerful indeed at the subjective
level.' It is not difficult to imagine that individuals who experience their
sexuality as a profoundly innate part of their being, and who feel no
sense of choice or control over the matter whatsoever, cannot *believe* in
social constructionist interpretations. This is because, to such individuals,
social constructionism simply does not make intuitive sense.

Social constructionist politics

However, the perception that social constructionism takes the ground
away from under the feet of the community has been challenged. To say
that homosexuality is socially constructed may seem the same as saying
that it is not 'real'. What it actually implies is that *no* 'identity' is 'real', in
the sense of existing independently of historical moment, culture and

socio-political context. As Vance suggests (1981: 16), 'To explain how reality is constructed does not imply that it is not real for the persons living it – or trivial, unimportant, or ephemeral.' Moreover, others have recognised that deconstructing deviations from any norm requires that we also deconstruct the norm itself. For example, if 'gay man' is a social construct, then so too is 'heterosexual man'. This may actually strengthen the demand for lesbian and gay human and civil rights, since it enables us to deconstruct *all* sexualities, and to ask *why* some are accorded higher social value than others. As Greenberg summarises (1988: 465):

> In demonstrating the historical variability of the cognitive categories through which people think about sex, this research undermines the seeming naturalness and objectivity of our own. Almost inevitably, it raises the question: if other times and places have been less repressive, why not ours?

He also argues that there is a straightforward moral argument for civil and human rights, which remains undiminished by accepting a social constructionist view: 'nothing in the social-constructivist position legitimates the denial of rights. Although it is well known that people can and sometimes do change their religious convictions, no one argues that people should be denied rights on the basis of their religion, or be forced to convert' (Greenberg 1988: 492).

Some have argued that social constructionism in fact offers a very strong basis for a rights movement, since it clears the way for collaboration with other marginalised groups. As long ago as the 1960s, some Black activist leaders in the US employed a similar approach in an attempt to form coalitions with homosexual rights groups (Altman 1993). More recently there have been attempts to form activist coalitions amongst transsexuals, sado-masochists, lesbians, gay men, bisexuals and others whose marginalisation springs from the social construction of their sexual or gender identity as deviant (Smyth 1992; Califia 1997).

Theoretical questions and developments

The political debate between essentialism and social constructionism within the lesbian and gay community will doubtless continue. There are theoretical questions, too, which social constructionists have still to answer.

The body

What part does the body and its limitations play in social construction? After all, it is one thing to demonstrate that 'lesbian' is a social construct, but it is quite another to conclude that a biological male can legitimately claim, on social constructionist grounds, that he is a lesbian, as some male students in American universities have done (Zita 1992). What, in this example, is the relationship between being a lesbian and being biologically female? If a biological man cannot be a lesbian, to what extent may we claim that 'lesbian' is *only* a social construct?

Performativity

In terms of gender and sexuality, social constructionism has led to the concept of *performativity*. Feminist academic Judith Butler coined the phrase, pointing out that if drag queens were 'performing' femininity, then so too were 'real' women. It is just as artificial, she reasoned, for biological women to dress up in 'feminine' garments, stagger around in high heeled shoes and paint their faces as it is when men do it (Butler 1990). The implication is that one person may perform, not one, but *several* genders.

Queer

Butler's thinking forms an important strand in an emerging academic discipline: queer theory. This multi-disciplinary perspective encompasses cultural studies, sociology, history, geography, literary studies, film theory, theology, music and art history. It is distinct from lesbian and gay studies, because queer theorists assume that heterosexuality requires critical study as much as homosexuality. Queer theory accords postive value to the ability to look at life from the perspective of a social outsider. Perhaps most significantly, since being 'queer' simply means that you refuse to take any forms of sexual and gender categorisation for granted, queer theorists are not all lesbians or gay men. They include bisexuals, transsexuals, transgender people, androgynous people and even queer heterosexuals (Smyth 1992; Seidman 1996; Califia 1997).

Criticisms of queer

This position is not universally accepted amongst the lesbian and gay community. Some lesbian feminists protest that deconstructing gender undermines arguments against the exploitation of women (Jeffreys 1990). Older activists tend to prefer the more traditional strategies of groups such as Stonewall, which makes use of tried and tested methods of political lobbying. The body has once more become a thorny question, with debate raging over whether a man who undergoes gender-reassignment surgery becomes a woman or something else, or whether a lesbian who takes testosterone in order to grow a beard is challenging sterotypes about lesbian masculinity or simply reinforcing them (Halberstam 1998; Kidd 1999). The more conservative members of the lesbian and gay community continue to call on essentialist theories of sexuality as the basis for their demand for equality.

Queer political activism has a carnivalesque aspect that springs from the attempt to live out the implications of social constructionism. The intention is a serious one – to demonstrate the instability of dominant constructs of sexuality and gender – but the playfulness of queer often alienates more conservative elements within the lesbian and gay community. It is important to recognise that such differences exist, and that there is as much diversity within that community as within the heterosexual mainstream. Just as it would be unacceptable to regard the behaviour of women watching a male strip show or men at a stag night as 'typically heterosexual', so there is no 'typically homosexual' way to behave.

Conclusion: implications for practice

To date, all attempts to prove an essentialist theory of sexual orientation have turned out to be underpinned by poor science. Indeed, at the time of writing, the press and media were reporting the failure of the 'gay gene' theory (*The Guardian*, 23 April 1999). However social theories are, by their very nature, not easily tested or empirically proven, and it is therefore unlikely that we will discover the 'truth' of social models of sexual orientation in the near future. Social constructionists argue that, since sexuality is demonstrably so flexible in response to social and cultural shifts, there is no one 'truth' to be discovered anyway.

From a social constructionist perspective we are able to explore the effect of social constructs on individual behaviour, whether conscious or unconscious. In addition, we are also able to follow this complex process a stage further, and examine the effects of individual behaviour on social constructs! This is interesting to sociologists, but from the point of view of those working in the health and social care professions, social constructionism offers two important insights.

Precisely because there is ample cross-cultural evidence to demonstrate the contingency of notions of homosexuality, the social constructionist critique of essentialist models of homosexuality has been particularly wide-ranging and thorough. The resulting body of evidence has led social scientists, such as Jennifer Terry (1997: 271), to conclude that 'we have voluminous evidence to show that science and medicine have played a big part in the making of homophobia'. The medical profession, and certain elements of statutory social care provision, have traditionally worked from a medical model of homosexuality, which is both essentialist and tends to pathologise, and this has inevitably influenced the relationship between the professions and those members of the lesbian and gay community whom they serve. Acknowledging this is an important first step in improving relations between practitioners and their lesbian, gay and bisexual clients.

Second, social constructionism tells us that the categories we use persist because they are, in the broadest sense, politically useful. This enables us to ask questions like: 'How does health and social care practice contribute to the social construction of sexualities?' and 'In whose interests is this being done?' It is clearly neither practical nor appropriate to enter into theoretical debate in the recovery room, radiography suite or case conference. However, the ability to ask such questions forms a key element of reflexive practice, and may make it easier for practitioners to introduce a new element of openness into their own thinking about sexuality. As such, it offers a firm foundation for the sorts of institutional change which user groups and researchers are increasingly demanding.

---

exercise

You can do this exercise on your own, or you can 'brainstorm' in a small group.

Write down a list of slang terms for 'gay man'. Make the list as long as you can, and do not worry if some of the words are offensive (they will be!). Now go through the list and mark every term that refers to anal sex. Then mark every term that refers to effeminacy. What does this tell you about the social construction of 'gay man' in your culture? What might the consequences of such a social construct be (1) for individual gay men, (2) for young men questioning their sexuality, and (3) for the attitudes of health and social care professionals?

You could follow this by trying a similar exercise with slang terms for 'lesbian', and see whether similar themes emerge.

Further reading

Altman, D. and others (1988) *Which Homosexuality: Essays from the International Scientific Conference on Lesbian and Gay Studies*. London: Gay Men's Press.

Caplan, P. (ed.) (1987) *The Cultural Construction of Sexuality*. London: Routledge.

Foucault, M. (1976) *The History of Sexuality: An Introduction*. Harmondsworth: Penguin.

Fuss, D. (1989) *Essentially Speaking: Feminism, Nature and Difference*. London: Routledge.

Nardi, P. and Schneider, B. (eds) (1998) *Social Perspectives in Lesbian and Gay Studies: A Reader*. London: Routledge.

Plummer, K. (ed.) (1981) *The Making of the Modern Homosexual*. London: Hutchinson.

Saraga, E. (ed.) (1998) *Embodying the Social: Constructions of Difference*. London: Routledge.

Seidman, S. (ed.) (1996) *Queer Theory: Sociology*. Oxford: Blackwell.

Stein, E. (ed.) (1992) *Forms of Desire: Sexual Orientation and the Social Constructionist Controversy*. London: Routledge.

Whisman, V. (1996) *Queer by Choice: Lesbians, Gay Men and the Politics of Identity*. London: Routledge.

6 sexual health

Introduction

Although an holistic approach to sexual health encompasses far more than the prevention and curative activities of genito-urinary medicine (GUM), sexually transmissible infections (STIs) remain at its core. The most serious STI is, of course, the human immunodeficiency virus (HIV), the agent responsible for the current global pandemic of acquired immune deficiency syndrome (AIDS). As we shall see, the social aspects of AIDS have contributed to the speed with which the virus established itself in different populations.

In this, HIV is not unique; similar social factors influence the distribution of all sexually transmissible infections. In order to promote sexual health, whether at an individual level or as a public health issue, it is necessary to understand both the biological factors of sexual transmission and the influence of socio-cultural factors. Accordingly, this chapter concentrates on the need to disentangle the effects that biological sex, gender, sexual behaviour and sexual orientation may have on sexual health, in particular the sexual transmission of infections.

The sexual transmission of infections

Sexual activity is a particularly intimate form of bodily contact, involving the partners in an exchange of fluids such as semen, saliva, sweat and the lubricating fluids of the vagina. It is therefore not surprising that it is a relatively efficient route for the transmission of those viruses, bacteria, fungi and other potentially pathogenic micro-organisms that result in the diseases that come under the heading of STIs. In the case of some diseases, such as hepatitis, sexual activity is only one of the modes of transmission whilst for others, such as gonorrhoea, it is the major or only known mode.

Some of the conditions associated with STIs, such as cervical cancer, syphilis or AIDS, are extremely serious. Others are inherently less so but may, if untreated, have distressing sequelae such as pelvic inflammatory disease or sterility. Some may be little more than an irritating nuisance in a healthy person but may cause more severe damage in an individual whose immune system is weakened by age, malnutrition, stress or other infections, such as HIV.

STIs are found world-wide and are extremely common (Llewellyn-Jones 1985; Porter 1997). Most sexually active adults are likely to experience some form of sexually acquired infection during their lifetime. Nevertheless, there are significant differences in individual vulnerability to infection and, as with every other kind of disease, these relate to social as well as biological factors.

Disentangling the biological and the social

Variations in the rate of STI infection between different social groups are largely due to social, cultural or structural factors rather than intrinsic biological differences. However, there is one important biological factor that influences vulnerability to STI infection, and that is the sex of those involved in a sexual encounter. The bio-logistics of STI transmission differ depending on whether sex is taking place between two men, a woman and a man, or two women. To understand this fully, we need to explore both the biology of transmission itself, and the influence of gender and sexual orientation. One of the simplest ways of doing this is to think of STIs as being transmitted either heterosexually or homosexually, and then to disentangle the additional factor of gender.

Heterosexual transmission: biological sexism?

Women are biologically more vulnerable to heterosexually transmitted infection than their partners. Doyal refers to this as 'biological sexism', concluding that:

> This 'biological sexism' . . . applies to most . . . sexually transmitted
> diseases . . . The reasons for this are complex but they derive partly
> from the fluid dynamics of unprotected sex, in which the male deposits
> several millilitres of potentially infectious semen over the surface of
> his partner's vagina, where it is likely to remain for some time.
>
> (Doyal 1995: 77–8)

Thus, we find that a woman is twice as likely to acquire gonorrhoea from
an infected male partner than is a man from an infected female partner,
whilst it has been estimated that women are anywhere from two to three
times more vulnerable to HIV infection during heterosex than are men
(Bury 1994; Doyal 1995).

The physical and social consequences of acquiring an STI are also
potentially more devastating for women than for men. Some infections
which are symptomless or trivial in men – such as trichomonas or chlamy-
dia – are potentially more harmful in women. Untreated infections may
spread upwards from the vagina into the cervix, uterus or fallopian tubes
and may give rise to pelvic inflammatory disease, scarring or blockage of
the fallopian tubes, ectopic pregnancies or infertility.

STIs in women may also go undiagnosed, or be diagnosed late. Often it
is less easy for women to recognise symptoms; a chancre that is obvious
on the tip of a penis may be less easy to spot when hidden inside the
vaginal entrance, especially when there is a cultural expectation that
women will be too modest to examine their own genitals. Moreover, the
continuing double standard of sexual behaviour may make it shameful or
embarrassing for women to seek treatment if they believe they have been
infected. In the case of HIV/AIDS, which retains some of its early associations with sexual promiscuity or deviance, general practitioners may be
slow to suspect HIV infection as a cause of illness in their 'respectable'
female patients (Panos Institute 1990; Wilton 1992; Berer with Ray 1993).

The social consequences of infection – particularly if it results in infertility
– may be devastating for women. In much of the world, women who are
known to have an STI, or who are unable to conceive, risk rejection by
their male partner, with consequent social exclusion and loss of income
(Panos Institute 1990; Patton 1994; Doyal 1995; Foreman 1999). In this
way, biological and social factors combine to make the risk of STIs very
different for women and men.

In terms of STIs and their potential consequences, therefore, heterosexual
activity poses a greater intrinsic risk to women than to men. Moreover,
Doyal's 'biological sexism' is combined with social factors that make it
extremely difficult for many of the world's women to exert any real
control over when they have heterosex, who their partners are and what
kinds of activities are involved (Gavey 1992; Doyal 1995; Wilton 1997a;
Berer 1998). Even in those parts of the world where women are accustomed to a great deal of sexual automony, social and cultural pressures
often restrict their choice in such matters. As one forthright young New
Zealand woman interviewed by Nicola Gavey recounted, 'if someone was
standing on my foot I'd fucking tell her . . . Someone's got their penis in

my vagina . . . and I don't feel able to ask them to stop. It's just *ridiculous'* (Gavey 1992: 26, emphasis in original). This 'ridiculous' situation becomes grave when activities which a woman feels powerless to resist may put her health at risk.

Women may also be poorly served by a medical profession that is too often sexist. Clinical discourse presumes the male body to be the norm, with the result that we have less information about women's health than we do about men's. Moreover, the medical 'gaze' has traditionally perceived women primarily in terms of their reproductive function, so that women's sexual health (as opposed to their reproductive health) has been a low priority relative to men's (Doyal *et al.* 1994; Berer 1998).

Homosexual transmission: safe sex?

If researchers have found that a combination of biological, cultural and social factors makes women more vulnerable than their male partners to heterosexually transmitted infections, a similar combination means that the risks of STI transmission between same-sex partners is very different. To state the obvious, sex between women does not involve semen. This is significant because semen offers a particularly effective medium of transmission for micro-organisms, including HIV. On the other hand, sex between men is likely to involve not one but two such deposits, thus increasing the statistical likelihood of transmission. For these most straight-forward physiological reasons, STIs are more prevalent among gay men than among lesbians (Shernoff and Scott 1988).

Research into lesbian sexual health confirms that sex between women is a generally inefficient route for the transmission of infections. Surveys have consistently found much lower rates of STIs among lesbians than among their heterosexually active peers (Boston Women's Health Book Collective 1989; Michigan Organization for Human Rights 1991; Dockery 1996; Institute of Medicine 1999) and evidence that HIV may be trans-mitted between women remains inconclusive (Bury 1994; Richardson 1994; Wilton 1997b). However, it does seem possible to transmit infections such as bacterial vaginosis between women and lesbian health activists quite rightly stress that *low* risk is not the same as *no* risk.

It is also important here to remember that sexual activity is not the same thing as sexual identity. In particular, just because a woman identifies herself as a lesbian this does not necessarily mean that she has no hetero-sexual experience. Some general practitioners, assuming zero heterosexual activity on the part of lesbians, have advised their lesbian patients that they do not need regular smear tests. However, studies have shown that the majority of lesbians have had sex with a man at some point in their lives, and recent surveys at lesbian sexual health clinics in London revealed abnormal smear test results among a significant minority of users (Farquhar 1999). The fact that sex between women is relatively safe does *not* imply that a lesbian *identity* offers protection against conditions associated with heterosex.

Although we now know that STIs are not as irrelevant to lesbians as was once believed, sex between women remains a relatively inefficient means for transmitting infections (Doyal 1995). This is not the case for men. Sex between men presents at least as much biological risk as heterosex, and may present specific additional risks. Heterosex generally involves semen being deposited in the body of the woman, not the man. Depending on the activity involved, it may be deposited in her vagina, anus or mouth, or outside the body altogether. The only significant physiological characteristic distinguishing sex between men from heterosex is that there is no vagina. Semen may therefore be deposited either outside the body or in the anus or mouth, potentially exposing both male partners to a level of risk similar to that borne by the female partner in heterosexual encounters. This factor contributed to the disproportionate impact of HIV on some gay male communities (King 1993).

Gender: is it different in homosex?

Given the extent to which gender socialisation and the structural inequalities between women and men permeate society, it is not surprising that they also have an impact on lesbians and gay men. It has, for example, been suggested that lesbians are more concerned with affection and intimacy than with sexual gratification, and that this is a product of traditional female socialisation unmodified in this case by sexual contact with men (Nichols 1988). By implication one might expect theorists to suggest that gay men, whose masculine socialisation is untrammelled by intimate association with women, would be more interested in sex, and more frequently sexually active, than their heterosexual counterparts. And, indeed, several writers have suggested just this (Shiers 1988; Kayal 1993; White 1997).

Such propositions cannot, however, be accepted at face value. In the first place, they often spring from a political agenda, being offered as 'proof' that homosexuality is unnatural and undesirable and that men's uncontrollable lust is meant to be tamed and controlled by the influence of women. For example, right-wing British philosopher Scruton writes:

> the promiscuous impulse of [men's] desires is neutralised and turned against itself when it is brought into contact with [women's]. And the self-regarding hesitations which poison [women's] are swept away by its contact with the insistence of [men's].
>
> (Scruton 1986: 308)

Feminist critics argue that it is precisely this kind of sexist reasoning which has led to the infamous double standard. For such reasons, many have challenged the notion that women are naturally sexless, innocent beings and that men are naturally promiscuous and predatory (Greer

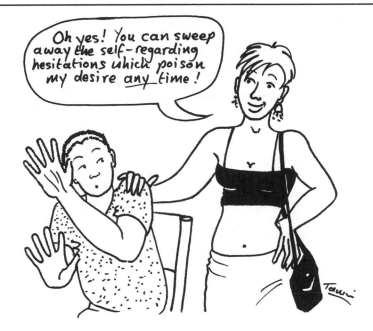

1970; Cartledge and Ryan 1983; Vance 1984; Segal 1994). The fact that this sexual 'division of labour' is not found in all cultures (Caplan 1987), nor in all periods of European history (Sawday 1995), combined with increasing evidence that it is shifting in contemporary European cultures, strongly suggest that the sexless woman and predatory man are very far from being universal human experiences.

Such evidence as does exist – and it is still very patchy – confirms that *most* of the lesbians who have been surveyed have fewer sexual partners than *most* of the gay men surveyed, that they are less likely to take part in casual sexual encounters and that they are more likely to place a high value on monogamy (Nichols 1988; Shernoff 1988; Smith 1992). However, it is not possible to draw any firm conclusions from this research. Samples have been relatively small and definitions of what counts as a sexual encounter remain problematic (Hunt and Davies 1991). Moreover, sex tends to be a lively topic of debate in lesbian and gay communities, and this can lead in turn to rapid shifts in sexual behaviour as certain practices go in or out of fashion (Nichols 1988; Califia 1994).

Community and risk

In order to understand the specific dynamics of gender within the lesbian and gay community, and to recognise its implications for sexual health, we need to examine the social and political importance of desire and sexual activity in the formation of lesbian or gay identities and subcultures.

Feminism

The relationship between political ideology and sexual behaviour is particularly evident in some lesbian subcultures, largely due to the influence of feminism. In the US and parts of Europe, many urban lesbian communities through the 1970s and 1980s experienced what came to be known as the 'sex wars' (for a fuller discussion see Wilton 1996). The issues were enormously complex but (risking simplification to the point of caricature) may be summed up as a split between two groups. One group (generally labelled revolutionary lesbian feminists) argued that pornography, sexual violence, rape, prostitution and sado-masochism were all elements of a patriarchal form of sexuality which disempowered women, and that, since lesbian sexuality offered women a refuge from patriarchy, lesbian communities should purge themselves of such behaviours (Hoagland 1988; Douglas 1990; Jeffreys 1990).

The second group (often called sex-positive feminists or sex radicals) argued that, since the oppression of women had historically included the repression of autonomous female sexuality, lesbians could empower themselves most effectively by exploring areas traditionally forbidden to women – including pornography, casual sex and sado-masochism (SAMOIS 1981; Nestle 1987; Califia 1994). Such differences are clearly likely to have consequences for individual lesbians' sexual and psychological well-being. Women who partake in a relatively restricted range of sexual practices may be exposed to fewer physiological risks than their more adventurous sisters. On the other hand, it is notoriously less easy to assess the impact on self-esteem and psychological well-being of sexual repression versus sexual fulfillment (SAMOIS 1981; Nestle 1987; Tiefer 1995).

Gay pride

Feminism is not the only political influence on lesbian and gay sexual behaviours and identities. The gay communities, which emerged in the post-Stonewall US and in Britain after the Wolfenden Report of 1957 and the partial decriminalisation of gay sex ten years later, had a newly confident attitude and took pride in being different from the heterosexual mainstream.

As autobiographical accounts of the time make clear, police activities prior to 1967 made the embryonic gay community a highly secretive environment, and one that many gay men were unaware of or unable to gain access to (Wildeblood 1955; Porter and Weeks 1991). For large numbers of gay men the only hope of finding affection, companionship or sexual intimacy lay in brief encounters in public places.

Sex under such circumstances was perforce very different from the kind that took place (or was popularly supposed to take place) between women and men. From the security of a legally and socially sanctioned marriage bed, in the comfort of an openly shared home, many heterosexuals held up their hands in horror at press reports of men finding sexual partners in public toilets or parks. Ignoring the fact that those involved had little choice in the matter, homosexual behaviour was seen as inherently degraded and base.

With the advent of the second wave of the women's movement in the 1960s it became increasingly difficult to maintain the rosy myth of marriage. New research exposed the despair which too often lurked behind the domestic facade; the extent of men's violence towards women in the home, including rape and sexual abuse; men's inability to offer intimacy and emotional support to their partners; and the sheer, soul-destroying tedium of life for suburban housewives (Coote and Campbell 1987; French 1992; Hague and Malos 1993; Doyal 1995; Bowker 1998). Suddenly it seemed as if the cosy, domestic world of sexual intimacy from which gay men and lesbians had been excluded for so long was not necessarily so desirable after all.

It is perhaps not surprising that some gay men began to believe that the lifestyles which had been forced on them when homosexuality was illegal offered a genuine alternative to the unhappy picture of marriage emerging from sociological research. They also sought to heal themselves and their communities of the guilt which was such a deep-seated part of gay experience for many. They did this by celebrating and reaffirming those elements of their sexuality that were most vilified: non-monogamous relationships and anal intercourse (Altman 1993; Wilton 1997a). The developing gay communities were also strongly influenced by the politics of the 'Sexual Revolution' of the 1960s, which promoted sexual exploration, non-monogamy and the pursuit of sexual pleasure as an element in the fight against materialist, militaristic, repressive lifestyles (see Greer 1970; Hansen and Jensen 1971; Neville 1971). By the 1970s, some sections of the rapidly growing urban gay communities of the industrialised West were developing a cultural and political life based on the belief that sex, and as much of it as possible, was both politically revolutionary and psychologically important.

AIDS: barriers to safe sex

Many gay academics and writers have commented on the tragic irony that the newly liberated, experimental sexual behaviour of these urban communities of gay men left them highly vulnerable to infection with STIs, including HIV (Altman 1986; Kayal 1993). However, it is not only amongst gay men that the spread of HIV has been encouraged by sexual and gender behavioural norms.

The fact that HIV continues to spread throughout the world highlights the extent to which sexual behaviour is mediated by social and cultural factors. It is not *easy* to become infected with HIV, only a limited number of specific behaviours carry the risk of transmission. Most activities that may be called 'sex acts' are incapable of transmitting HIV or are extremely unlikely to do so. The list of 'safe' sexual activities is much longer than the list of 'unsafe' ones, and includes a wide variety of behaviours ranging from the most low-key to those enjoyed only by a minority with specialised tastes. The most risky activities are those involving penetration of the vagina or anus with a condom-less penis, leading long-time AIDS commentator, Cindy Patton, to summarise her safe sex advice as 'don't get semen in your anus or vagina'.

This throws into the foreground a particularly sharp distinction between the biological and the social. Biologically speaking, nothing could be easier than safe sex. Human ingenuity is more than a match for a virus, which demands such specific behaviours for its transmission. However, *socially* speaking, the practice of safe sex is extremely difficult. The majority of sex acts carry little or no risk; only penile penetration is dangerous. However, this is also the single sex act that carries the greatest significance in all cultures. Depending on the social, cultural and religious context, non-penetrative sex may be regarded as immature, as 'not real sex', as no more than foreplay, as perverted or kinky, or even as sinful.

Gender is also a significant factor. In many cultures, the only route to adult status and economic security for women is through motherhood and, as we have seen, women often lack the power to control sexual encounters (Doyal *et al.* 1994; Doyal 1995; Heise 1997; WHO 1995). Adult masculine status is similarly bound to erection, penetration, ejaculation and/or paternity as proofs of potency – a situation often described as 'phallocentric' – and safe sex may therefore appear emasculating to heterosexual men. So, although it is technically easy to avoid the sexual transmission of HIV, in socio-cultural terms it is dauntingly difficult.

The gay plague myth and its consequences

Many (although not all) of the earliest cases of AIDS that came to the attention of the US medical profession were young gay men, and it was therefore assumed that the new syndrome was in some way a direct consequence of the urban gay lifestyle. Physicians variously named it gay-related immune deficiency (GRID) or 'gay cancer' (Shilts 1987). In Britain, the tabloids dubbed it the 'gay plague' (Watney 1987). In a climate of general homophobia, this unlikely theory appeared credible. It also meant that those stricken with this terrifying new disease faced blame and rejection when they most needed sympathy and care.

For a long time it has been evident from WHO surveys that the overwhelming majority of instances of HIV transmission globally – up to 80 per cent – result from condom-less heterosex (WHO 1995). In much of the US, HIV disease has been the leading cause of death of women of childbearing age since the mid-1980s. Yet gay plague myths retain a powerful hold on the imagination.

This is perhaps not surprising; such myths offer someone to blame, they enable 'ordinary' people to believe that their ordinariness keeps them safe, and they act to reinforce existing forms of social exclusion. Moreover, they are publicly endorsed by those in power, as this statement from Sir Alfred Sherman, co-founder of the Centre for Policy Studies, demonstrates:

> AIDS is a problem of *undesirable minorities* – mainly sodomites and drug abusers, together with numbers of women who voluntarily associate with this sexual underworld.
>   (*Independent on Sunday* 1 November 1994, added italics)

Sherman's comments were made at a time when it was generally known that such views were mistaken, yet his powerful position lent renewed credibility to the notion that AIDS is a disease of sexual deviance in general and homosexuality in particular.

Hindsight enables us to recognise that this misperception gravely hindered early attempts to control the epidemic, since it drew attention away from those who were *not* gay men. Destitute people and drug users in the US had been dying through the 1970s from something dismissively referred to as 'junkie pneumonia'. A Danish doctor, Margrethe Rask, died in 1977, having been ill for several years with a mysterious collection of symptoms, which her friends initially put down to overwork (Shilts 1987). Other such isolated cases were being picked up in many countries around the world. Had the US medical profession remained more open-minded about what was going on, important links between these cases *might* have been made much sooner than they were. This might have made it possible to recognise at a much earlier stage that we were dealing with an infectious agent, rather than some bizarre consequence of 'fast lane' gay lifestyles, which heterosexuals could safely ignore.

A further consequence relates to the nature of medical research in the US. The Centers for Disease Control (CDC), whose staff were the first to suspect the existence of the new syndrome, is located in the richest country in the world, and has access to the most advanced medical research community and some of the most generously funded clinical establishments. It should have been a stroke of luck for humanity that the new disease came to the attention of the medical profession in the US.

Unfortunately, the US is also one of the most homophobic cultures in the Western world (Pharr 1988; Schulman 1994; Deitcher 1995). Those prejudices, which led doctors to interpret AIDS as the results of a gay lifestyle in the first place, then ensured that those struggling to set up research programmes received no government funding (Patton 1985; Shilts 1987; Kramer 1990; Kayal 1993). Initial research was funded entirely by voluntary donations from the gay community, and *all* AIDS-related services – including telephone help lines, drop in centres, social care services for the sick and counselling for the bereaved – were set up by gay voluntary groups. As Philip Kayal recounts:

> When not using their own money to assist needy sufferers, these early 'volunteers' and their friends stood outside discos and gay bars soliciting donations for research. In just three months they donated $11,000 to the Kaposi Sarcoma Fund established at New York

University Medical Centre. By mid 1982, they were able to give nearly $50,000 more to individual doctors, social workers and hospital research centres.

(Kayal 1993: 2)

Fifty thousand dollars is an enormous amount to fund-raise outside gay bars, but it is very little in medical research funding terms. The US government steadily refused to fund *any* research into AIDS because the close association of the disease with homosexuality made it politically unwise for the Republican administration to be seen to offer any help. The political battles over AIDS, battles which have squandered time, energy and resources, can all be traced back to the initial assertion by doctors that the disease was gay-related, and led Mathilda Krim, director of the CDC, to call AIDS 'the epidemic that was allowed to happen' (Wilton 1992). The socio-political consequences were disastrous.

First, those who were not gay-identified were reassured that 'normal' people had nothing to fear from the new disease, since it was the result of a deviant lifestyle. This undoubtedly hampered attempts to promote safer sex. Although it is impossible to guess the numbers involved, it is likely that many thousands became infected heterosexually during this period of denial.

Second, although it was soon recognised that 'normal' heterosexuals *were* vulnerable to AIDS, this did not mean that the 'gay plague' theory was thrown out. Rather, gay men were blamed for the appearance of the disease *amongst heterosexuals*. If this was a gay disease, ran the argument, then it must be passed on to heterosexuals by bisexuals or by drug users sharing needles with gay men. This led to an upsurge of homophobic rhetoric and violence.

This was particularly so in the US, where right-wing activists and evangelical fundamentalists called for the extermination of homosexuality. Community centres, churches and bookshops were firebombed, AIDS grafitti appeared everywhere, lesbians and gay men were the victims of beatings, acid attacks and shootings, bricks were thrown through their windows (Patton 1985; Altman 1986; Carter and Watney 1989; Kramer 1990; Kayal 1993; van der Vliet 1996).

The perceived link between HIV and homosexuality meant that any attempt to control the epidemic, whether by clinical research, sex education in schools, promoting safer sex or providing proper services to those already infected, met with a hostile response. Although Britain has not seen the extremes of homophobic violence witnessed in the US, attempts to control the spread of HIV initially met with very similar kinds of resistance. Safer sex education in schools, it was claimed, would prompt pupils to experiment with homosexuality, providing clean works would encourage drug abuse, and making condoms available in prisons would condone sodomy (Watney 1987; Aggleton *et al.* 1990).

Many outspoken public figures, both in Britain and the US, showed *more* concern to promote a particular version of sexual morality than to prevent further sickness and deaths (Shilts 1987; Aggleton *et al.* 1990; Wilton 1992; Kayal 1993; King 1993). At this early, crucial stage in the pandemic, such social and political factors were a significant obstacle to infection control and disease prevention.

Conclusion

We have seen that, because of the fluid dynamics of sexual intercourse, HIV and other STIs pose a greater risk to those (both women and men) who are sexually active with male partners. Social and cultural factors, especially gender, may also result in unequal vulnerability to infection. This is seen very clearly in the context of the HIV pandemic, where the initial readiness to interpret AIDS as a consequence of homosexuality resulted in heterosexual denial at every level. In the final analysis, this was one of the reasons why the epidemic continued to spread so rapidly through the populations of the West *after* an effective means of prevention had been identified. Clearly, effective sexual health promotion requires a full understanding of the social and cultural influences on individuals of different gender and sexualities.

However, disease is not the only health hazard associated with sex and sexuality. In order to understand fully the links between sexuality and health we need to explore some of the complex issues which surround sexual identity, and that is the subject of the following chapter.

---

exercise

You can do this exercise on your own, but it does work best if several people do it together. If working alone you will need paper and pen/pencil. If working in a small group it helps to have a pad of stick-on notes.

1 Think of as many sexual activities as you like (kissing, bondage, masturbation, etc.) and write each one on a slip of paper or a stick-on note. Be explicit and use your imagination, you should be able to come up with at least a dozen!

2 Arrange them in order, from those that carry LOW RISK of HIV transmission to those which carry a HIGH RISK. Think carefully about each activity; exactly *how* might it result in the transmission of HIV?

3 You should end up with a large number of activities at the LOW RISK end. Those at the HIGH RISK end should only be ones where semen is deposited in one partner's anus or vagina. Look at the activities that ended up as LOW RISK. What kinds of activity are they? How are they generally regarded? What are the implications for people's ability to adopt safer sex practices?

4 Now arrange the activities in different categories depending on whether they may be carried out between TWO WOMEN, between TWO MEN, or between A WOMAN AND A MAN. You may wish to

devise some way of representing your categories in diagram form; perhaps by drawing up three columns, or by sketching overlapping circles, or by means of separate boxes. Again, think carefully about each activity and what it involves before deciding which category to assign it to.

5 What happened when you tried to do this? What does this tell you about the sexual practices of lesbians, gay men and heterosexuals? Did anything emerge which surprised you, or which you had not thought of before? What are the implications for safer sex promotion?

Further reading

Fitzsimons, D., Hardy, V. and Tolley, K. (eds) (1995) *The Economic and Social Impact of AIDS in Europe*. London: Cassell/National AIDS Trust.

Foreman, M. (1999) *AIDS and Men: Taking Risks or Taking Responsibility?* London: Panos Institute and Zed Books.

King, E. (1993) *Safety in Numbers: Safer Sex and Gay Men*. London: Cassell.

Moore, O. (1996) *PWA: Looking AIDS in the Face*. London: Picador.

Panos Institute (1990) *Triple Jeopardy: Women and AIDS*. London: Panos Institute.

Wilton, T. (1992) *Antibody Politic: AIDS and Society*. Cheltenham: New Clarion Press.

The best way to keep up to date on treatment issues is to subscribe – or get your library to subscribe – to Gay Men's Health Crisis *Treatment Issues* newsletter. For subscription information write to: GMHC, Treatment Issues, 119 West 24th Street, New York, NY 10011, USA.

7 writing sexual orientation into health

Introduction

There is broad agreement amongst health and social care professionals that an holistic concept of 'health' must incorporate a sexual dimension (Aggleton 1990). Sexuality can have a powerful impact, whether positive or negative, on individual health and well-being. It can also influence our ability to function successfully in society.

The impact of gender on women's health has been the subject of several decades of research and, more recently, researchers have become concerned with its consequences for men. However, such research often fails to identify the consequences of heterosexuality, and it is now becoming clear that this can lead to a lack of clarity in defining research objectives, and may even result in failure to identify specific health hazards.

The impact of homophobia on physical and mental health is rightly receiving much greater attention. However, the health consequences of being lesbian or gay are not necessarily negative. Lesbian and gay respondents in several studies have scored higher than their heterosexual counterparts for measures of self-esteem, satisfaction with life and other positive psychological variables (Isay 1989). Other studies have shown generally good levels of psychological well-being amongst those lesbians and gay men who are open about their sexuality (Clark 1987). As we have seen, lesbians are also less likely than their heterosexually active counterparts to suffer from sexually transmitted diseases, and this is likely to have generally beneficial consequences for health and well-being.

Clearly, sexual orientation may influence physical, emotional, psychological and social health in a variety of ways, many of which are as yet under-researched and poorly understood. This chapter offers an overview of what is known, and suggests important ways in which sexuality needs to be 'written in' to health and social care research.

Health, well-being and sexual identity

It is difficult to gather information about the relationship between sexual identity and health. Homophobia makes it unsafe for most individuals who are lesbian or gay to make their sexuality known to health care providers and heterosexist assumptions mean that some of the negative health consequences of homosexuality may be exaggerated, whilst others may be ignored. On the other hand, the health hazards of *heterosexuality* itself have seldom been recognised. Researchers in all disciplines are only just beginning to recognise and account for the bias that heterosexism and homophobia may introduce into their work (see Wilton 1995), and accounting for such bias still requires an unusual awareness and a conscious shift in perspective.

Risk and sexual identity: breast cancer

It is often difficult to disentangle sexual identity from other influential factors in terms of risk. To take one fairly typical example; there has been much discussion within lesbian communities in the US and the UK about the question of breast cancer. There has been a suggestion that lesbians are at greater risk of acquiring breast cancer than non-lesbian women, and this has naturally caused anxiety and concern (Wilton 1997b; Institute of Medicine 1999). A critical look at the research findings that have been used to underpin such arguments reveals just how difficult it can be to isolate sexual identity in this way.

It seems fairly certain that breastfeeding offers significant protection against breast cancer, and that both obesity and excess consumption of alcohol appear to increase the chances of developing the disease. The link between breast cancer and lesbians has then been constructed by arguing that (1) lesbians are less likely than non-lesbian women to have children and (2) there are relatively high rates of alcoholism and obesity among lesbians (Kerner 1995). However, these extrapolations need to be treated with some scepticism. First, we simply do not know what proportion of lesbians have children and methodological problems mean that this situation is unlikely to change in the near future. Even if we could prove what percentage of lesbians are mothers, it is still childlessness, not being a lesbian, that increases the risk of breast cancer. The protective factor – breastfeeding – remains the same whatever your sexual orientation.

There are slightly different problems with research findings which seem to indicate that lesbians are more likely than non-lesbian women to be obese or to abuse alcohol. For those who experience homophobia on a daily basis, it is recognised by many researchers that obesity and substance abuse are likely consequences (see essays in Shernoff and Scott 1988; McClure and Vespry 1994), since they are closely associated with stress (Doyal 1995). In addition, it is difficult for lesbians to relax and socialise in most of the leisure facilities that heterosexuals take for granted and they are entirely dependent on the (unpredictable) tolerance and good will of the heterosexual majority for their personal safety in public spaces. The 'gay villages', which have grown up in many towns and cities, offer a modicum of safety for those who wish to socialise in peace, but this kind of safe space is closely associated with the consumption of alcohol. Many researchers have suggested that this in itself contributes to the disproportionate levels of alcohol abuse found in some surveys (Shernoff and Scott 1988; Petersen 1996; Institute of Medicine 1999).

However, even the finding that lesbians are disproportionately likely to suffer from obesity and alcoholism is based on small samples, which are unlikely to be representative. There is a very real possibility that those women who comprise a sample population are more likely than the 'average' lesbian to have problems with alcohol and obesity, simply because they are more likely to be 'out', or to participate in the community culture based in bars and clubs, from which samples are likely to be recruited.

The increase in breast cancer risk which seems to be associated with obesity and heavy drinking should certainly concern those lesbians who fit these categories. However, there is no evidence that a lesbian who is obese or drinks heavily is at greater (or lesser) risk than a non-lesbian woman with a comparable history of obesity or alcohol consumption. In other words, lesbianism is once more not the significant risk factor.

It must be concluded that lesbianism does *not* increase the risk of breast cancer. However, it would be reasonable to suggest that behaviours which do increase the risk of breast cancer are likely, for a range of reasons, to play a different part in the lives of lesbian and non-lesbian women. This means that efforts to reduce rates of breast cancer should incorporate research activity designed to increase our understanding of these complex issues, so that *all* women may be given information appropriate to their circumstances.

Questions of stress: the evidence

> From the shit on the door to greet me when I arrived home at night to the dangerous vandalism of my car and the desecration of my garden and fences, to shouting and banging on windows to frighten my daughter and her teenage babysitters, and the endless verbal abuse, we lived life under siege . . .
>
> (Lesbian living in Yorkshire,
> cited in Mason and Palmer 1996: 40)

From accounts such as this, we might expect homophobia to be a significant factor in conditions such as hypertension, heart disease, alcohol and substance abuse, anxiety, depression, suicide, irritable bowel syndrome, immune disorders and other stress-related conditions. Researchers have hardly began to investigate the health consequences of homophobia, but findings to date indicate that there is much to learn (Muir-MacKenzie and Orme 1996; Sheffield Health 1996; Institute of Medicine 1999; Mugglestone 1999). We know, for example, that lesbians and gay men are at disproportionately high risk for suicide and attempted suicide (Trenchard and Warren 1984; Whitlock 1988; Herdt 1989; Nicholas and Howard 1998) and for alcohol and substance misuse (Hall 1993). Findings such as these demonstrate the need for more research into homophobia as a factor in stress-related ill health.

Heterosexuality: now you see it, now you don't

One important consequence of heterosexism is that more attention is paid to the potentially harmful consequences of a lesbian or gay lifestyle than to those associated with heterosexuality. This is partly because a 'heterosexual lifestyle' is seldom thought of in these terms, and its health effects tend to be discussed purely in terms of gender. This can make it difficult to isolate the influence of heterosexuality itself.

After three decades of research into gender and health there is substantial evidence that a heterosexual lifestyle can be detrimental to women's mental and emotional well-being. The physiological risks sometimes associated with heterosex – such as infections, bruising, minor trauma to tissues and local irritation or pain – are well documented, and are probably taken for granted as a fact of life by most heterosexually active women (Boston Women's Health Book Collective 1989; Doyal 1995). In those cultures that demand female genital mutilation, or the insertion of herbs into the vagina to tighten it in the interests of the male partner's pleasure, such practices contribute to physical trauma for the women involved (Walker and Parmar 1993; Wilton 1997a).

In addition, women who are heterosexually active must deal with the reproductive potential of heterosex. Either they face the possibility of pregnancy which, even when desired, carries its own quota of health risks or they must use some form of contraception. With the exception of methods that rely on abstinence during the fertile days of the woman's cycle, all forms of contraception carry some health risks (Boston Women's Health Book Collective 1989). The health hazards associated with contraception are generally thought of as a generic 'women's' health issue, but it is important to acknowledge that they are a consequence of heterosexual activity, rather than biology alone.

However, the failure to take sexual orientation into account can cut both ways. For example, the risks of pregnancy and childbirth are usually linked unproblematically to a heterosexual identity, despite the fact that a significant number of lesbians are biological mothers (Saffron 1996; Griffin and Mulholland 1997). This general failure to distinguish between sexuality and gender results in a rather unsophisticated approach to certain aspects of health research, and means that the data collected is often less useful than it could be.

Male violence: who is at risk?

One of the most significant findings of feminist research has been the extent of domestic violence (Brownmiller 1975; Smart and Smart 1978; French 1992; Hague and Malos 1999). There has been much discussion of late about partner abuse in lesbian couples (see, for example, Lobel 1986; Renzetti 1992), and of the abuse of men by their female partners. Nevertheless, around 90 per cent of domestic violence is perpetrated by men on women (Doyal 1995; Bowker 1998), and researchers have suggested that 'the true rate of men *ever* beating a wife or female lover in the life of a relationship is close to 50 per cent for all couples' (French 1992: 190). Concluding a summary review of the literature, Marilyn French (1992: 190) writes that, 'In the United States, a man beats a woman every twelve seconds, and every day four of these beatings reach their final consummation, the death of the woman.'

Of course, women are neither the only nor the most frequent victims of male violence; men are most often violent towards other men. Indeed, violence of all kinds seems to be largely a male problem, for those charged with or convicted of crimes of violence are disproportionately men, and arguments continue as to whether this is due primarily to biological or social factors (Connell 1987; Bowker 1998). For women, therefore, the risk of violent assault increases with the frequency or closeness of their contact with men. This strongly suggests that heterosexual activity and/or a heterosexual identity may make women more vulnerable to this kind of assault.

Lesbians are probably as vulnerable as non-lesbian women to a different form of violent assault, stranger rape. However, studies have shown that most rapes are carried out by boyfriends, husbands and other men known to the victim. Lesbians may therefore be less at risk from this form of assault, simply because their social and intimate lives tend to include fewer men. However, lesbians may experience other forms of violence, such as gay-bashing, precisely because of their sexuality. Clearly, there are good reasons for suggesting that both sexuality and gender influence the degree of risk and the kind of assault most likely to be experienced by different groups.

Domestic bliss?

It seems that sexual orientation may impact on health in quite complex ways, although this may not be recognised by researchers. This is certainly the case in one area about which we have quite detailed knowledge, long-term heterosexual partnerships. The unequal status of women and men means that, around the world, women's physical and mental health sometimes suffers as a direct result of marriage and domestic responsibilities (Morgan 1984; Brekke *et al.* 1985; Panos Institute 1990; Doyal 1995; Macionis and Plummer 1997).

In the majority of heterosexual households around the world, women's well-being is constrained by the heavy burden of domestic labour and by the expectation that the male members of the household are entitled to a greater share of resources, including food (Panos Institute 1990; Doyal 1995; Foreman 1999). Despite moves towards greater equality in some industrialised nations such as Britain, women still outnumber men as full-time carers of babies and young children and as carers of adult dependants such as chronically sick or disabled family members and the frail elderly (Payne 1991; Graham 1993; Richardson 1993) and are responsible for a disproportionate share of routine domestic labour (Malos 1980). To this unhappy picture must be added the damaging emotional consequences of routine or unpleasurable heterosex. As Lesley Doyal concludes;

> many women derive little pleasure from heterosexual practices that prioritise male wants. Lack of desire can itself be a source of distress and low self-esteem . . . it is clear that coercive sex can be a significant cause of anxiety or depression. 'Routine' sex too may be an important but largely unrecognised element in the complex of factors that leave so many women with little sense of autonomy or self worth.
>
> (Doyal 1995: 63)

Several studies (for example, Bernard 1972) have concluded that marriage enhances men's well-being but damages women's. Bernard went so far as to write of a 'housewife syndrome', with a range of anxiety symptoms including 'nervousness, fainting, insomnia, trembling hands, nightmares, dizziness and heart palpitations' (cited in Doyal 1995: 37). It is widely accepted that there is a close association between being the full-time mother of young children and being clinically depressed (Brown and Harris 1978; Ussher 1991).

What part does sexual orientation *per se* play in this depressing scenario? Evidence is patchy. For example, some pioneering work carried out at the London School of Economics suggests that at least some lesbian households are able to achieve a degree of equity in child-rearing, which seems supportive of the mental health of both partners (Dunne 1997, 1998), but no longitudinal studies have yet been completed. Some heterosexual couples are quite consciously trying to establish more egalitarian partnerships (VanEvery 1996), although researchers who study such relationships have often found that change is slow in coming:

> my evidence shows that it is difficult for women to make cohabiting [hetero]sexual relationships equal. Not only is it rare for men to be committed to equality, but even when they are, the process is a struggle.
>
> (VanEvery 1996: 50)

More research is needed if we are to discover how the unequal status of women and men affects the domestic lives of lesbians, gay men, bisexuals and heterosexuals, and what impact this has on the well-being of these different groups.

Gender or sexuality? New questions

Unpicking gender and sexuality is, as we have seen, a difficult task. By examining the findings of research into lesbian well-being and comparing these with existing information about non-lesbian women, this section demonstrates one possible method for isolating the effects of sexual orientation on well-being. This is followed by a discussion of masculinity, and its impact on the health of gay and non-gay men.

Lesbian mental well-being

A broad range of research has established beyond question that heterosexuality carries risks to women's health. It is less easy to state with any degree of certainty how well lesbians compare with their heterosexual sisters in similar circumstances, although the availability of relevant data is increasing. The greater degree of equality between lesbian partners that has been observed (Cossis Brown 1992; Dunne 1997) might be expected to have health benefits, but this has not yet been explicitly demonstrated. Other studies have concluded that lesbians generally have a more positive orientation towards the labour market than non-lesbian women, leading to an unusual degree of autonomy and satisfaction with paid employment (Dunne 1992, 1997).

Against positive findings such as these must be set the stresses of dealing with homophobia in the workplace (Levine and Leonard 1985; Hall 1992), and the added difficulties of living in a relationship that is not sanctioned by the state. So it is not yet possible to make a direct comparison between heterosexual women and lesbians when considering the impact that sexual orientation may have on mental health.

Nevertheless, it is important to recognise that many of the mental health stressors, which are often assumed to be common to 'women' as an undifferentiated category, are in fact a consequence of *heterosexuality* for women. Given the quantity of evidence that depression and anxiety in women is closely associated with elements of the heterosexual lifestyle, more work remains to be done to assess the extent to which lesbian lifestyles may *protect* women from these factors. We simply do not have enough information to decide whether the damage done to lesbians' health by homophobia is outweighed by the benefits of a non-heterosexual lifestyle.

Machismo: gay or straight?

It should by now be clear that researchers have not been asking all the right questions. Because heterosexuality is so unquestioningly taken as the norm of human behaviour, the many and complex links between gender, health and illness are seldom analysed in terms of sexuality. For example, it is well known that young men during the years of early adulthood are statistically at high risk of dying as a result of accidents or violence (see Figure 7.1).

These statistics are commonly interpreted in the light of stereotypical adolescent male activities such as over-use of alcohol, drunken driving, pub brawls, 'joy riding', football hooliganism, etc. One of the most important consequences of feminism has been that researchers have begun to

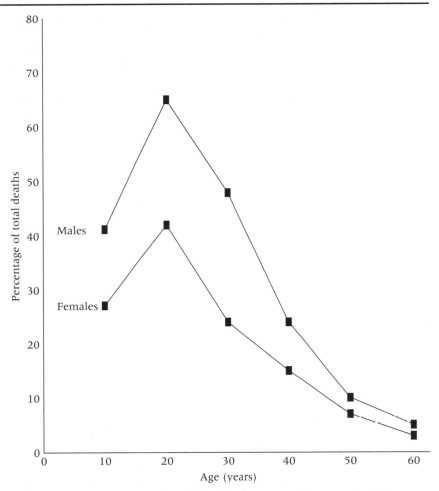

Figure 7.1 Percentage of total deaths due to accidents and violence. *Source:* Simplified from OPCS, *Trends in Mortality*, 1978.

examine the social construction of masculinities, and the extent to which men are compelled to demonstrate their masculinity in ways that are ultimately self-destructive or dangerous, such as being violent towards women or other men or treating sex as a competitive activity (Reynaud 1981; Connell 1987; Stoltenberg 1989; Davidson 1990; Giddens 1992; Bowker 1998).

Historically, the ultimate duty of a man to the nation-state has been in his role as a soldier prepared to lay down his life to defend his country. The social construction of masculinity appears to retain vestigial elements of this role, even in peacetime. Young men, the argument goes, have to prove their manhood by risk-taking; drinking too much, driving too fast, winning fights with other men and having sex with as many women as possible. The stereotype of 'men behaving badly' is a familiar one, and undoubtedly does play a major part in the death and injury rates among young adult men.

Again, what is missing in most of these discussions is the part played by sexual orientation. Almost all critical theorists of masculinity recognise that one of the ways in which 'real men' prove their manhood is by rejecting anything associated with homosexuality or effeminacy (Reynaud 1981; Connell 1987; Davidson 1990; Simpson 1994).

This is complicated by recognising that the social construction of masculinity does not, and cannot, impact solely on men who happen to be heterosexual. Indeed, some gay male theorists debate its influence on the personal development of individual gay men or on the development of gay male subcultures (Dyer 1989; Gough 1989). Nevertheless, there has not, as yet, been any empirical research that links these two key points and which would enable us to say that a heterosexual identity *per se* is either dangerous to or protective of men's health, although there is clear agreement that something called 'masculinity' is. As Formani comments, 'whatever masculinity is, it is very damaging to men' (Formani 1991: 13).

Homosexuality and mental health

For decades, homosexuality was itself defined as a mental illness. As empirical support for this position collapsed under the weight of contrary findings, mental health professionals were forced to respond accordingly, but did so with considerable reluctance. The American Psychiatric Association only removed homosexuality from its official list of mental disorders (the DSM) in 1973, a decision which was followed in 1975 by a statement of support from the American Psychological Association.

These decisions were not supported unanimously by all members of the Associations, and there is still a significant minority of psychiatrists and clinical psychologists who insist that homosexuality is either an illness *per se*, or symptomatic of mental disturbance (Gonsiorek 1988). Indeed, a vestigial element of the illness model of homosexuality remained until 1987, when the diagnosis of 'ego-dystonic homosexuality' (conflict or distress about one's homosexual feelings) was finally removed from the DSM. As recently as 1995, the London School of Psychotherapy was the target of angry protests when Professor Charles Socarides, a leading American proponent of the mental illness model of homosexuality, was invited to speak (Powell 1995), but his is a largely discredited view.

The mental health professions in the developed world no longer regard lesbians and gay men as sick. However, this does not seem to have resulted in the mental health system offering a sensitive service to lesbian and gay users. On the contrary, many mental health professionals seem to have retained homophobic attitudes and many of their lesbian and gay clients report inadequate or distressing experiences in consequence (Annesley 1995; Davies and Neal 1996; Jackson 1998). In response, a gay-affirmative strand of mental health service provision is slowly developing (Clark 1987; Davies and Neal 1996). Mental health professionals are increasingly interested in the varying strategies used by lesbian and gay individuals to cope with social hostility, and the different outcomes of these strategies in terms of self-esteem and well-being. Homophobia, rather than homosexuality, is now identified as the major problem for most gay people.

Homophobia

The mental health implications of homophobia may be terrifyingly direct. Around the world, many thousands of lesbians and gay men risk death on account of their sexuality, and, as we have already seen, homophobic violence is characterised by its extreme nature. The 'respectable' and widespread nature of homophobia means that it crosses class, cultural and ethnic lines and that there is no automatic safety even in your own family. A black teenager who experiences racist abuse or assault will at least find support and safety in their own family and community; this is not necessarily the case for a young lesbian or gay man, many of whom meet with abuse, hostility, rejection or violence from their own family members (Trenchard and Warren 1984; Whitlock 1988; Comstock 1991; Evans 1996).

Anna Durell recounts the story of a young woman who called London Lesbian Line for support because, 'she had been admitted to hospital with concussion and a fractured arm when her father had thrown her down-stairs after she told him she was a lesbian' (Durell 1983: 15). Organisations that work with homeless people are slowly beginning to recognise that young lesbians and gay men are often thrown out by their families when their sexual orientation becomes known, and that they make up a significant proportion of the young homeless (Greater London Council 1985; Evans 1996; Stoneham Housing Association 1996).

It is not surprising therefore that researchers have identified the hostility and rejection of family members as particularly harmful to the mental and emotional health of lesbians and gay men. For some, the pain is compounded by the attitude of politicians, public figures, the press and even members of the helping professions. Some lesbians and gay men in crisis or distress may meet rejection and hostility wherever they turn for help and understanding. Experiences such as these are qualitatively different from the mindless hostility of gay-bashing. As one clinical psychologist puts it:

> Irrational hatred and abuse can be understood when it comes from socially damaged people who are trying to vent blind anger. But when the wounds are inflicted by family, friends, trusted counsellors, and civic leaders, the wounds go deep and damage self-esteem. A scarred and seriously damaged self-concept is the result.
>
> (Clark 1987: 92)

If such characteristics of homophobia distinguish it from other forms of oppression such as racism, another distinctive factor is that lesbians and gay men are not easily recognised by their appearance. The outrageously dressed drag queens and leather-clad bikers who march on Gay Pride parades or appear in films or on television are not representative of the daily self-presentation of most lesbians or gay men. Whatever popular folk wisdom may hold about always being able to 'spot one', it is generally only possible to recognise an individual's sexual orientation if they want you to.

Safe in the closet?

This may appear to offer a degree of protection, but the sense of security that comes from this invisibility is very much a false one. Many gay activists have commented wryly that tolerance of homosexuals would arrive much more swiftly if every lesbian or gay man in the land turned purple overnight and it was realised how 'normal' most of the community are. In this sense, the inability to detect homosexuals enables homophobia to flourish unchallenged.

It is for other reasons, however, that the ability of lesbians and gay men to 'pass' unnoticed in daily life can be damaging. Anyone who passes as heterosexual in daily life is exposed to the unthinking homophobia of those around them. At times this may be amusing. Gay journalist and radio presenter Nigel Wrench tells the entertaining story of what happened when he and his producer, David Cook (also gay), went to interview Mary Whitehouse for a programme on gay rights:

> when she spoke of a meeting in the Seventies, and how 'obvious homosexuals' barracked her and threw what seemed to be blueberry tarts at her, I asked how she could pick out the 'homosexuals'. It was apparently all their outfits. David and I stole a quick look at each other's Levis, but we remained unrumbled. We didn't tell her we were gay.
>
> (Wrench 1998: 11)

Occasions such as this may become the stuff of in-jokes between the people sharing the experience, but overhearing even casual and unthinking anti-gay remarks made by individuals who *in fact* would never consider assaulting anyone may be very frightening indeed (Mason and Palmer 1997).

Moreover, concealing such a significant part of one's self takes an obvious psychological toll. As one long-time gay activist put it:

> We pulled the ugly green frogskin of heterosexual conformity over us, and that's how we got through school with a full set of teeth. We know how to live through their eyes. We can always play their games, but are we denying ourselves by doing this? If you're going to carry the skin of conformity over you, you are going to suppress the beautiful prince or princess within you.
>
> (Harry Hay 1979, cited in Thompson 1994: 186)

Understandably, concealment and secrecy may contribute to the burden of stress borne by individuals who are lesbian or gay. Case evidence from the clinical practice of gay-affirmative mental health practitioners, combined with empirical research findings, suggest disproportionately high rates of anxiety disorders, clinical depression, alcohol and substance misuse, chemical dependency and other indicators of psychological distress (Shernoff and Scott 1988; Erwin 1993). There is also a substantial body of evidence for relatively high rates of suicide and attempted suicide, especially among lesbian and gay young people (Trenchard and Warren 1984; Erwin 1993).

One large American study was carried out in 1977 involving over 5000 lesbian and gay respondants, aged 14–82 years. Of this sample, no less than 40 per cent of the men and 39 per cent of the women had attempted or seriously considered suicide (Jay and Young, cited in Erwin 1993). Of course social attitudes towards lesbian and gay people were more rigid in 1977, but later studies have continued to report comparable findings, with recent research suggesting that the risk of suicide among adolescent lesbians and gay men is from three to six times as great as for their heterosexual peers (Remafedi *et al.* 1991; Erwin 1993; Nicholas and Howard 1998).

Although homophobia has been clearly identified as a major factor in the extremes of psychological distress suffered by many lesbians and gay men, this troubling situation remains largely ignored. 'These data', Erwin concludes, 'point to high levels of emotional distress among gays and lesbians.' But, she continues, 'Although homosexuality is increasingly becoming a topic of academic research and debate, there is a noticeable paucity of reference to gay suicide in the public health and mental health literature' (Erwin 1993: 439, 448). There is, for example, no mention of the high rates of lesbian and gay suicide in *Health of the Nation* documentation relating to the drive to reduce suicide rates across the UK.

Conclusion

Although researchers have tended to ignore its significance, there is strong evidence that sexual orientation *is* an important influence on mental and physical health and well-being. The pressures of maintaining a heterosexual masculine identity, the consequences for women of an inequitable heterosexual lifestyle, the often traumatic pressures on lesbians and gay men of homophobia and the additional stressors of sexism for lesbians are all detailed in the literature.

The implications of this for practitioners of health and social care are enormous. First, these findings lend powerful support to a social model of health. They indicate that social factors, rather than purely medical ones such as genetic predisposition or biochemical malfunction, are of primary significance in the genesis of physical illness and psychological distress. This implies that, as the World Health Organization acknowledges (Naidoo and Wills 1994), well-being can neither be enhanced in individuals nor promoted throughout societies without instigating social change. From the existing evidence, it is clear that discrimination on grounds of sexual orientation has as much potential for harm as more widely recognised prejudices such as racism.

The second implication is that the health and social care professions, which have too long unthinkingly contributed to the pathologisation and marginalisation of lesbians and gays, have a responsibility to take homophobia and its consequences more seriously than has been the case to date. There is a need for research programmes designed to isolate the effects of sexual orientation (whether positive or negative) from those of gender, and for existing data to be reinterpreted without heterosexist bias. In the context of professional demands for research-based practice, it is time to put questions of sexuality high up on the research agenda.

---

exercise

Think about the detailed elements of your own area of practice. How would you describe the characteristics of your client group? What kinds of problems do they come up with, and what is your role in their care? What kind of relationship are you able to form with them? Using the information in this chapter, try to indentify the possible significance of (1) gender, (2) sexual activity and (3) sexual identity in relation to each of the factors you have described. Are there issues which you have not thought about before? What steps might you take to strengthen your own practice in this area?

Further reading

Institute of Medicine (1999) *Lesbian Health: Current Assessment and Directions for Future Practice*. Washington, DC: National Academy Press.

Mason, A. and Palmer, A. (1996) *Queer Bashing: A National Survey of Hate Crimes Against Lesbians and Gay Men*. London: Stonewall.

Muir-MacKenzie, A. and Orme, J. (eds) (1996) *Official Report of the 1996 Conference: Health of the Lesbian, Gay and Bisexual Nation*. Plymouth. The Harbour Centre, 9/10 Ermington Terrace, Plymouth PL4 6QG.

Petersen, K.J. (ed.) (1996) *Health Care for Lesbians and Gay Men*. New York: Haworth Press.

Royal College of Nursing (RCN) (1992) *Health of Half the Nation*. London: RCN.

Shernoff, M. and Scott, W. (eds) (1988) *The Sourcebook on Lesbian/Gay Health Care*. Washington, DC: National Lesbian and Gay Health Foundation.

Wilton, T. (1997) *Good for You: A Handbook on Lesbian Health and Wellbeing*. London: Cassell.

8 sexuality and the family

Introduction

The family is an important arena of professional intervention both in health care and (perhaps especially) in social care. It is therefore important to have some insights into the origins of 'the family' and into the variety of family structures that exist. In terms of sexuality, too, the family is a crucial concept, since it is a key element in the policing of sexualities.

However, contemporary notions of what constitutes 'a family' reflect a historical process of development, which did not stop once it got to the nuclear family of two adults and 2.4 children. This chapter gives a brief overview of the history of the changing family, discusses its importance in health and social care, and outlines its significance in terms of the social organisation of sexuality. It continues by examining some current debates; the threat to 'family values', the social construction of motherhood and the problem of male sexuality in relation to fathering.

Sexuality, care and the family

The political and professional frameworks within which care is delivered are grounded in a particular set of assumptions about what the family is, what it should be and what part it plays in the well-being of individuals and of society. Many aspects of statutory social service provision are designed to strengthen, or temporarily stand in for, elements of family support that are absent or failing. Social workers may be assigned to families experiencing problems, may take children away from those families seen as inadequate or damaging, and may offer support to those whose natural families are unable or unwilling to provide it. In many senses, social work may be seen as an institutionalised attempt to compensate for the drawbacks of the nuclear family type when faced with the changing needs of an advanced industrialised society (Connell 1987).

The Welfare State

The original aims of those who set up the British welfare state are becoming increasingly costly to realise, due to demographic and political changes. Demographic changes include increased life expectancy and growing numbers of older people as the baby boomer generation ages. Political factors include the global recession following the oil crisis of the 1970s, monetarist economic policies aimed at withdrawing the safety net of welfare, and multi-national companies shifting production from the industrialised West to third world countries, where labour is very cheap (Ham 1992). These and other factors have caused severe strain on welfare provision.

Welfare has always been delivered in a 'mixed economy', involving four sectors: the public or statutory, the private or commercial, the voluntary or charitable, and the domestic or informal. Of these, the domestic sector has always provided by far the greatest proportion of care, since it is within the family unit that most of us receive the bulk of our health and social care throughout the lifecycle (Hart 1985; Giddens 1992, 1997).

Social scientists agree that, among other things, 'the family' is a political concept, subject to intervention on the part of the state (Connell 1987; Richardson 1993; Giddens 1997). This has become more explicit in recent years, partly as a result of the monetarist policies of Conservative administrations in the 1980s and 1990s. These policies promoted a highly idealised notion of the family and the emotions invested in it, partly in order to defend massive cuts in public services (Smith 1994; Stacey 1997)

This shift back to the family or 'community' as welfare provider causes particular problems for women. As many critics point out, although care in the family is presented as a gender-neutral concept, it usually means care by female family members. Although a significant proportion of care is provided by men, the overwhelming bulk of care for young children, adult family members, the chronically sick, disabled and elderly is provided by women in their familial roles of wife, mother, daughter and daughter-in-law (Baldwin and Twigg 1991; Payne 1991; Graham 1993; Langan 1997). Moreover, reductions in the welfare 'safety net' did more than simply place greater economic and social burdens of care on to families. The attempt to lock the family more firmly into the mixed economy of welfare went hand in hand with attempts to regulate the *kinds* of family that people could form. More legislation targeting reproductivity and sexuality was passed at this point in British political history than at any previous time, and such legislation had the effect of sanctioning a particular notion of what a family *should* be (Weeks 1991; Smith 1994).

By their very nature, legal changes of this kind are closely associated with health and social care provision, since it is through the health and social services infrastructure, as well as the education service, that state agencies get access to families. These areas of professional practice are, therefore, inevitably implicated both in regulating families and in promoting particular ideas about what a family is. 'Especially in poor and working-class families, state agencies and reformers seeking to eliminate deviance regulate personal and family life through the work of professional experts' (Andersen 1988: 152). It is important for those working in HSC to be able to recognise the social control element of their professional practice and to exercise a degree of personal judgement over this aspect of their role, in line with the model of the reflexive practitioner.

A history of the nuclear family

Social historians disagree about whether or not the 'nuclear family', consisting of a 'nucleus' of father, mother and the biological offspring of both of them, developed as a direct consequence of the Industrial Revolution. However, there is general agreement that the growth of industrial capitalism encouraged the idea that the home should be a sanctuary – at least for men – from the public world of paid labour. This led to certain key beliefs about gender, including the notion that the 'ideal' family should consist of a male bread-winner, earning enough to support a home-bound wife, whose task it was to maintain the family home and its other occupants. At earlier periods in European history, when families had to be self-sufficient economic units, this arrangement would have made little sense (Ziegler 1979; Giddens 1997).

Victorian values

The great social reform movements of the Victorians hastened this transformation of family lives. The new way of life gave middle-class women very little opportunity to develop a sense of meaning or of self-worth, since all they had to do was to give the servants their instructions. Some fell victim to mental health problems or chronic physical symptoms, giving rise to the stereotype of the fragile, fainting Victorian woman quite at odds with the heavy work carried out by the majority of working-class women below stairs or in the factories or mines (Bassuk 1985; Showalter 1987). Some middle-class women became philanthropists, visiting the sick or the poor, and laying down the roots of professions such as health visiting, community nursing and social work. Others became politically active, many in the struggle for universal suffrage or in the fight against slavery, and others as social reformers intent on improving the lives of the poor.

Since the great social reformers (men as well as women) came from this class, they took it for granted that the forms of family that they had experienced were the best. Not surprisingly, the reforms that they set in motion aimed to enable poor families to build for themselves a copy of the middle-class way of life, which soon took on the status of a desirable norm:

> beginning in the nineteenth century and continuing through the present, the concept of the family, as it originated in the well-to-do classes, extended through other strata of society . . . the concept of the family as we know it today – a privatized, emotional, and patriarchal sphere – has its origins in the aristocratic and bourgeois classes.
>
> (Andersen 1988: 150)

It would be difficult to overstate the significance of this for the social organisation of sexuality, for gender roles and for the eventual development of the welfare state. The 'ideal' family promoted by the reformers was also strongly supported by the Church, in an attempt to sustain religious values, and this had consequences that were felt around the globe. Victorian colonialists and missionaries tried to root out the cultural values of the societies that they exploited. Where the social organisation of sexuality and reproduction differed from the Victorian middle-class norm, it was often proclaimed as evidence of the savage, child-like or animal-like nature of the indigent peoples, and efforts were made to 'civilise' them by forcing them to adopt Western habits of modesty in dress, monogamous heterosexuality, Christian marriage and a domestic division of labour (Ware 1992; McClintock 1995).

There was no place in the Victorian bourgeois family for anything other than reproductive heterosexuality, and a profoundly gendered heterosexuality at that. With men given access to the public sphere and women increasingly confined to the home, the social construction of male and female sexuality became polarised. Men were seen as having uncontrollable sexual lusts, whilst (white, middle-class) women were seen as the 'angel in the home', free from erotic feeling and driven instead by a deep-seated maternal instinct, which led them to tolerate sexual intercourse only in the interests of reproduction (Hobson 1987; d'Emilio and Freedman 1988).

Modern social reformers who recommend a return to Victorian values seldom recognise that there was a dark and troubling side to sexuality in this era. Women who were sexually active were seen as less 'civilised' or (in the Darwinian model popular at the time) less 'evolved'. Prostitutes were seen as a necessary evil, offering a 'seminal drain' (Treichler 1988) as an outlet for male lust, whilst women who were working-class, black, mentally ill or lesbian were often characterised as sexually insatiable (Miller 1995; McClintock 1995). Child prostitution was not uncommon. A common lay health belief was that intercourse with a virgin child would cure venereal disease, and special brothels were set up for this purpose, often employing orphans or 'idiot' girls and sometimes providing infected male clients with girl children as young as six (Smith 1979).

A lasting legacy

Victorian ideas about sex and gender, especially the notion of the sexless 'good' mother and her opposite, the sexually active 'bad' mother, have had lasting consequences for health and social care. It has been suggested that the tolerance afforded to men's sexual adventures, on the other hand, may have been one of the social factors leading to the highly problematic relationship between some men, children and sex with which we are struggling today (Connell 1987; Heise 1997).

Bad mothers, good mothers and sex

Even today, there is much anxiety about sex in association with mothering. Some of this is based on Freudian notions such as the so-called 'primal scene' of intercourse between mummy and daddy (popularly believed to traumatise any child unfortunate enough to witness it), the incest taboo, and the dark undercurrents of the Oedipus and Electra complexes (for critical discussion, see Merck 1993; de Lauretis 1994). Since Freud, most of us now take it for granted that familial relationships contain a dangerous erotic element, which must be controlled.

However, the idea of the sexless mother did not originate with Freud. Rather, it was Victorian familial ideology which insisted that women lacked sexual desire. Women's desire was for children, and they tolerated sexual contact with their husbands only because they longed for children. Desire was therefore constructed as the *opposite* of the maternal 'instinct'. These beliefs lingered well into the twentieth century. Brandt (1989: 28) comments that, 'many doctors presumed that most women were sexually anaesthetic . . . this apparent lack of interest in sex among women was typically cited as an aspect of their moral superiority'. He goes on to cite the words of one medical doctor published in America in the early years of the twentieth century: 'There are but few . . . hopeless sexual perverts. The vast majority have no very pronounced sexual feelings and a majority are altogether deficient in this respect.'

'Sexual anaesthesia' was the hallmark of the kind of woman to be entrusted with the task of caring for innocent children. Fatherhood, in contrast, was associated with no such celibate leanings. Men's sexual 'drives' and 'urges', although regarded as base, were assumed to be the natural and necessary expression of masculinity, and since their pure and wholesome wives could not be expected to put up with such baseness, the answer clearly lay in prostitution (Wells 1982; Hobson 1987; d'Emilio and Freedman 1988).

Sexually transmitted infections – then known as venereal diseases – were a serious problem. Many women were infected, and were often unable to fulfil their maternal duties as a result, since infection could lead to sterility and/or the birth of infected and sickly children. Philandering men were blamed for bringing disease home to their innocent wives, but it was women sex workers who were most directly stigmatised. After all, men were behaving quite 'naturally' when they had casual extramarital sex, whereas the women they had sex with were not:

> Prostitution is pregnant with disease, a disease infecting not only the guilty but contaminating the innocent wife and child in the home with sickening certainty almost inconceivable; a disease to be feared as a leprous plague, a disease scattering misery broadcast, and leaving in its wake sterility, insanity, paralysis, and the blinded eyes of little babes, the twisted limbs of deformed children, degradation, physical rot and mental decay.
>
> (Victorian tract, cited in Brandt 1989: 32)

This gothic catalogue of horrors is laid at the door of the prostitute, and at its heart lies anxiety about preserving the purity of motherhood.

A minor, but vital, ingredient in this anxious discourse of sexuality was the figure of the lesbian. Because homosex is non-procreative, lesbian desire represented a particular challenge to the notion that women endured sex only in order to get children. Even today commentators note that one reason why there is such a moral panic about lesbian mothers is that lesbianism is, by definition, a *sexual* identity; 'the characterization of lesbians as nonprocreative beings . . . render[s] the image of the lesbian mother shocking and disconcerting . . .' (Weston 1993: 158).

As records of Parliamentary debates indicate, the notion of female sexlessness lead to the assumption that 'normal' women were far too innocent to think of something as disturbingly erotic as lesbianism all by themselves. One peer insisted that lesbianism should not even be mentioned in legislation, in order to preserve the innocence of women:

> It would be made public to thousands of people that there was this offence; that here was such a horror . . . Is there any necessity for it? How many people does one suppose are really so vile, so unbalanced, so neurotic, so decadent as to do this? . . . you are going to bring it to the notice of women who have never heard of it, never thought of it, never dreamed of it.
>
> (Saraga 1998: 179)

This extract is from the 1920s, but such attitudes continue to have implications today, perhaps especially for midwifery. As the authors of one midwifery textbook suggest:

> it was always felt that for a mother to be sexually active was against the dominant definition of motherhood as an almost pure and unsullied state . . . [But] if motherhood is the desire of all 'natural' and 'real' women, how does one explain the lesbian mother? Either lesbianism is a part of being a 'natural' woman or motherhood is not, this is the inescapable and logical dilemma posed by a rigid definition of femininity and motherhood.
>
> (Symonds and Hunt 1996: 118–19)

This brief foray into the complex issues of motherhood has demonstrated that anxieties about the family, the nation state and social control are tightly bound up with the figure of the mother, and that the 'good mother' is defined against a range of 'bad mothers', whose badness is *because* they are sexually active. Clearly the relationship between motherhood, female sexualities and the family is both extremely complex and highly charged.

Fatherhood: men, children and the spectre of the paedophile

Masculinity and femininity are constructed as polar opposites, so that what men are, women are not and vice versa. Many scholars who have studied the social construction of gender suggest that the social and psychological pressure on men to disassociate themselves from anything feminine is particularly strong (Connell 1987; French 1992; Heise 1997; MacInnes 1998). To be a 'real' man is to be as different from women as possible, and to be seen as such. Masculinity must not only be done, it must be seen to be done:

> the crucial thing about being socialized a male, being masculine, is not to be like a girl. That's what they learn. Not so much to be like a man – except they're taught never to show emotion – but *never* to be like a girl. So masculinity is not being feminine.
>
> (Interviewee in Arcana 1983: 89)

We might therefore expect 'fatherhood' to be constructed as somehow the 'opposite' of motherhood, and some writers have suggested that this is indeed the case (Symonds and Hunt 1996; Giddens 1997). In contrast to the intimate, affectionate and nurturing role associated with mothering, the dominant construct of fatherhood is characterised by responsibility for the economic support of the family unit and by authority within the family. This means that boy children are socialised into an outward-looking, employment-orientated and emotionally detached role, which fails to equip them for intimate emotional relationships, whether with their own children, their sexual partners or their friends. The consequences of this have been identified as distressing and frustrating both to women and, increasingly, to men themselves (Reynaud 1981; Stoltenberg 1989; Davidson 1990; Giddens 1992).

The socialisation of men also seems to result in specific forms of sexuality. In summary, this has been described as goal-directed, competitive, instrumental, mechanistic, emotionally detached and irresponsible (Connell 1987; Stoltenberg 1989; Davidson 1990; Giddens 1992; Miedzian 1992; Heise 1997). Several male academics, gay and straight, have pointed to the potentially damaging consequences that this may have for gay male sexuality, unmodified as it is by the presence of female sex partners with contrary socialisation (see, for example, Giddens 1992, but for a summary see Edwards 1994).

Others have pointed to possible links between this social construct of masculine sexuality and child sex abuse. The sexual abuse of children is usually, although not exclusively, abuse of girls by their more powerful male relatives – fathers, stepfathers, uncles, grandfathers and sometimes older brothers (French 1992; Giddens 1992; Heise 1997). The widespread nature of child sex abuse remained hidden until researchers in the late 1960s and early 1970s began to uncover evidence that it is disturbingly common. Particularly troubling have been claims that the perpetrators display few, if any, traits of psychological abnormality: 'Psychologists have tested men imprisoned for rape and incest and find them "normal"' (French 1992: 198).

Despite substantial evidence that it is 'ordinary' men in 'ordinary' families who abuse, two groups of men have been made scapegoats in public discourse; gay men and paedophiles. The homophobic assumption that gay men 'recruit' underlies the often expressed hostility to permit them to parent or care for children (see below). There is also an assumption that paedophilia, a relatively rare form of personality disorder characterised by exclusive and extreme sexual interest in children, represents the *greatest* risk to vulnerable children.

Psychologists, such as Sayce and Perkins (1998: 16) point out that, statistically, the mentally ill paedophile is *not* the man that most children have cause to fear:

> The huge family outcry over the whereabouts of released child rapists/ murderers obscures the fact that most child rape/assault occurs within families. Where is the similar outcry – the demonstrations demanding that children are protected from . . . fathers, uncles, brothers?

At the time this statement was published there had been several mass demonstrations, notable for their ferocity, by parent groups trying to prevent convicted paedophiles from being housed in their area on release from custody. Such public scapegoating of convicted paedophiles is understandable. However, it leaves unanswered important questions about how best to protect children, given that most child rapists are neither homosexuals nor paedophiles, but otherwise 'normal' men, assaulting their own children.

Furthermore, some studies have shown that such men may see nothing wrong with their behaviour. Andersen, for example, concludes that 'the father/assailant feels no contrition about his behaviour . . . fathers did not . . . express nurturing feelings for the victim or understand the destructiveness of the incest' (Andersen 1988: 173).

This has led some to conclude that, rather than concentrating only on the mentally ill, those who wish to halt the sexual abuse of children must turn their attention to the unwanted consequences of a masculine socialisation that grew out of the Victorian value system (French 1992; Heise 1997).

Mad, bad and dangerous to know?

These Victorian 'family values' also underpin the contemporary construction of lesbians and gay men as unnatural, sick people devoid of the normal, decent 'instincts' of heterosexuals. Indeed some have suggested that, since any dominant group requires people who are 'other' in order to clarify its own boundaries, the demonisation of homosexuality was a necessary prerequisite to establishing the normative status of heterosexuality (Stacey 1997). As Reid writes (1995: 190), 'In familial discourse the production of "family" as desirable norm has always required freaks and outcasts that name the norm indirectly by virtue of their departure from it'.

Lesbians and gay men, along with sex workers, child molesters and others, were not only excluded from the construction of 'the family', but became identified with its opposite, seen as in some sense 'anti-family'. This, too, has had important implications for the practice of health and social care. Reid concludes:

> from the latter half of the nineteenth century and down to the present, psychiatrists, experts of all kinds, and the media have constructed narratives of middle-class households also 'endangered' by wayward hysterical mothers and daughters, effeminate sons, unmarriable cousins, sexual 'perverts', emancipated women, and maniacal or impotent fathers.
>
> (Reid 1995: 190)

Of course vulnerable people do need protection from the kinds of abuse that may occur in families. However, some scholars argue that the effort directed towards protecting the abstract *idea* of 'the family' has damaging consequences for individuals who are unable or unwilling to conform to this rather limited model of living (Weeks 1985, 1991; Kaufmann and Lincoln 1991; Weston 1993; Smith 1994).

Family values: always in crisis?

There are those who believe that the traditional family is now in decline, and statistics certainly seem to support this position. In the United States as well as Britain and across mainland Europe, divorce rates are rising, along with other suggestive indicators such as births out of wedlock and the number of single parent households. In Britain we have become accustomed to hearing politicians utter dire warnings about the social consequences of family instability in general and lone parenthood in particular, pointing to rising crime rates, increased truancy from schools and a deepening drugs problem (Reid 1995; Giddens 1997).

Various social groups have been publicly made scapegoats for the perceived crisis in the British family. Working-class families, immigrants from the Indian subcontinent, African-Caribbeans of the post-Windrush era, travellers and Romanies have all been seen as creating 'problem' families. Lesbians and gay men have been singled out for particularly vicious public attack, since they have been accused not just of incompetence in family life but of being the *enemies* of the family.

Such notions both reflect and, to a great degree, depend on medical discourses of normality and naturalness. Hartouni, for example, cites British infertility expert Patrick Steptoe, who finds it, 'Unthinkable . . . Willingly creating a child to be born into an *unnatural situation* such as a gay or lesbian relationship' (Hartouni 1997: 25, my emphasis). An authoritative statement such as this is a clear example of what Mort (1999) terms 'medico-moral politics'. Steptoe's position clearly has implications for lesbian and gay families' access to sympathetic health care, but also contributes to public anxieties about a lesbian and gay community, which is both ever-growing and out to destroy the 'normal' family. This is not just the stuff of dubious stand-up comics, nor is it restricted to the religious right in the US. Such views have been expressed quite openly in local authority meetings and on the floor of Parliament, and have appeared in legal statute and other official documents.

The homosexual threat

In December 1986, the leader of South Staffordshire Council, Councillor Brownhill, came up with a public health strategy in response to the HIV pandemic; he proposed, on the record, that 90 per cent of gay men should be exterminated in gas chambers. A peaceful local protest which followed was broken up by police and the members detained in jail over the Christmas break, after which they were released without charge. Councillor Brownhill received no reprimand from any quarter, nor did he at any time offer an apology or retraction. His words came shortly after the *Daily Express* had demanded that 'homosexuals . . . should be locked up. Burning is too good for them. Bury them in a pit and pour on quick lime' (all cited in Baaden 1991: 122–3). In the House of Commons, speaking during a debate on the Human Fertilisation and Embryology Act in support of a proposed clause prohibiting lesbians from receiving fertility treatment, Conservative MP David Wilshire declared that:

> Our society is based on long-term commitments between adults in a
> family setting. It is based on a child having a mother and a father,

and on the importance of family life . . . Our social standards are *deliberately being undermined*, and it is high time for those of us who think that that is wrong to stand up and say, in words of one syllable, that we shall fight that decline and prevent it going any further.

(Smith 1994: 212, my italics)

There was an attempt to prevent lesbians and gay men from fostering children by including a paragraph in the 1989 Children Act, which instructed social services departments that 'the chosen way of life of some adults may mean that they would not be able to provide a suitable environment for the care and nurture of a child'. Of course, vulnerable children should not be fostered in unsuitable environments. However, the text goes on to state that ' "Equal rights" and "gay rights" policies have no place in fostering services' (Smith 1994: 211).

Perhaps the clearest official signal that lesbians and gay men were to be regarded as a threat to the normal family came in 1988 with the passing of Section 28 of the Local Government Act. This Section, which gave rise to huge demonstrations across Britain and mainland Europe, reads as follows:

2A – (1) A local authority shall not – (a) intentionally promote homosexuality or publish material with the intention of promoting homosexuality; (b) promote the teaching in any maintained school of the acceptability of homosexuality as a pretended family relationship.

As legal experts were quick to point out, the law is unworkable; it is not possible to reach a legally enforceable definition of what it means to 'intentionally promote homosexuality' (and it is, in any case, absurd to imagine any local authority doing any such thing). Moreover, the passage referring to schools is meaningless, since the Local Government Act does not apply to them. Indeed, the Department for Education was obliged to write to all headteachers explaining that they should take no notice of the new law (Colvin and Hawksley 1989). Nevertheless, it remains the *only* British law to have actively and selectively discriminated against an identified social group. As such, Jack Cunningham, speaking as Minister for the Cabinet Office in 1999, described it as 'wrong in 1987 . . . wrong in 1999' (Stonewall 1999: 6).

This continuing demonisation of homosexuality must be seen as a consequence of the tendency to promote a particular type of family as normal and proper. It has become an intrinsic part of the struggle to define and police familial behaviour. As Reid (1995: 185) comments, ' "Family" has always been an alibi if not a licence for visiting social others with unremitting violence.'

Writing in 1945, sexologist Thomas Moore warned of the danger posed by homosexuality to the family and the state. He uses both the language of disease and the social-scientific concept of subcultural formation to produce a confused but highly emotive picture of homosexuality as a kind of *social epidemic* with grave consequences for all, and concludes that 'The growth of a homosexual society in any country is a menace, more or less serious, to the welfare of the state' (Moore 1945: 57).

Same old story?

How much truth is there in the idea that the traditional family is under new kinds of threat? Sociologists often use the term 'cereal packet family' to refer to the stereotypical norm of a 'traditional' household. This phrase describes the situation where:

> There are two parents, aged between 20 and 45, legally married to each other, and not having been married to anyone else previously. Two children, born of these parents (and not others), live with them. The husband's work is a priority and, even if the wife has work, it is part-time or interrupted by child-rearing and does not form part of a career. The wife takes on the bulk of the household tasks even if the husband may help occasionally . . . Lastly, its members are happy.
>
> (Abercrombie *et al.* 1994: 272)

Not only does this imagery fail to reflect increasing diversity in family norms but, as Abercrombie *et al.* point out, 'it is doubtful if such images ever accurately described the majority of families in Britain'. The 'traditional' family is no such thing. Social history and anthropology make it plain that different forms of family structure evolve in response to the different environmental and social demands of different geographical environments

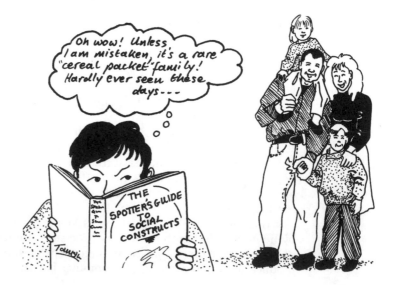

and different historical eras. Family forms develop, become obsolete and are replaced with new forms over time. Such changes may be imperceptibly gradual; very simple cultures may retain a family structure that is appropriate to their way of life for hundreds or thousands of years. On the other hand, changes may be relatively swift; where social change is rapid then family forms must adapt in response.

Any change in family form will itself inevitably contribute to wider social change. During the First and Second World Wars, for example, women were recruited into the labour market in huge numbers. At this time, nurseries were provided to care for their children and the working mother was portrayed as a responsible and good citizen. When the fighting men returned home needing work, women were urged back to the home, nursery provision was withdrawn, childcare experts pronounced that 'maternal deprivation' was a dire threat to the well-being of infants and working mothers began to be portrayed as *irresponsible* and selfish (Martin 1987).

Though changes of this kind are inevitable, they are likely to be experienced by many people as threatening. Since the current 'ideal' family is one where we expect to have our most intimate and basic needs met, it is perhaps not surprising that the prospect of change provokes anxiety. But the threat to family life perceived by many commentators is far from unique to our age. It is clear that conservative elements in European societies have always feared what seems to be an inevitable process of change and development. 'The cry "death of the family"', writes Reid (1995: 191), 'is a time-worn refrain almost two centuries old'.

The family as building block of the nation

Any threat to family stability is often presented as making society as a whole vulnerable to outside threat or internal collapse. A report published by the US government in 1993 warned that:

> The family trend of our time is the disinstitutionalization of marriage and the steady disintegration of the mother–father child raising unit . . . No domestic trend is more threatening to the well-being of our children and to long-term national security . . . fragmentation of families poses a threat to the nation.
>
> (Cited in Reid 1995: 184)

The heterosexual nuclear family has long been closely identified with the strength and security of the nation state. Reid compares the words of twentieth-century President Roosevelt, 'we cannot as a Nation get along if we haven't the right kind of home life' and nineteenth-century French politician Guizot, 'The family is now more than ever the first element and last bulwark of society' (187, 189). Still more explicit are the sentiments of Sarah Hale, whose domestic manual *Manners: or, Happy Homes and Good Society* was a best seller in 1869:

> But one race retains the Eden laws of love and home; and in that
> race only is the faith and the worship of the true God. From that race
> were the families that settled and made our American people. In two
> centuries and a half, this North American empire has gained power
> and place in the great family of nations: compared with her, those
> old cradles of civilization and centers of knowledge and glory – Asia
> and Africa – are now only blanks in the lot of humanity.
>
> (Hale [1868] 1972: 24)

Nationalism, religion, notions of racial supremacy and national security
all contribute to Hale's ideal family type. These nineteenth-century ideals
remain so powerful that contemporary politicians are able to use them
today to manipulate public opinion about events that may have little to
do with family policy. When, for example, US President Clinton nominated
an openly lesbian candidate to a government post, moral majority spokes-
man Jerry Falwell sent the following mailing to supporters, asking for
donations:

> President Clinton's nomination of Roberta Achtenberg, a lesbian, to
> the Department of Housing and Urban Development is a threat to the
> American family . . . Achtenberg has dedicated her life to winning
> the 'rights' of lesbians to adopt little babies. Please help me stop her
> nomination.
>
> (Cited in Stacey 1997: 461)

Falwell's campaign is a clear example of the deliberate exploitation of
homophobia for political ends, which is such a feature of public life in the
United States (Signorile 1993; Schulman 1994; Deitcher 1995; Stacey
1997). The political landscape in Britain is very different. Nevertheless, as
long as the social and political infrastructures of the nation state remain
so closely bound up with a particular form of family, the state is likely to
obstruct the development of alternatives. As Reid concludes:

> Weak and vulnerable as it was constructed and as it is still portrayed
> today, the normative family and its healthy bodies nonetheless stood
> in the eyes of many a politican, charity worker, and public health
> officer as the pillar of society and the sole barrier standing between
> social order and anarchy.
>
> (Reid 1995: 189)

The cry 'family in danger!', far from being new, has been the traditional
accompaniment to the processes of social change in complex societies. By
itself, this insight does little to remedy the problems suggested by ever-
increasing divorce rates, rising number of single parent families and spiral-
ling crime statistics. However, sociologists of the family point out that the
conclusions generally drawn from such statistics may be misleading. The

next section discusses some of the changes that appear to be taking place in family structures.

Changing families and pretended families

Divorce rates are increasing in the industrialised world. People are also tending to marry later (although there are significant class differences), and rising numbers of infants are born out of wedlock – as many as one in four in Britain (Richardson 1993). The cereal packet family is becoming rare:

> today, sociologists are hard put to locate the domestic family and its human bodies anywhere . . . Something like less than 14 per cent of households in the United States fulfill the old domestic norm . . . the figure drops to 5 per cent if the additional factor of never having been married before is thrown in
>
> (Reid 1995: 192)

In Britain, politicians have tended to hold divorce and lone-parent families responsible for a wide range of social problems from drug abuse to falling educational achievement and rising inner city crime. However, evidence from Sweden (where half the babies born are to unmarried mothers and where 29 per cent of children live in lone-parent families) suggests that such links are misleadling. 'Research in Sweden' writes Giddens (1997: 155), 'turns up little sign of the problems fatherlessness is supposed to bring in its wake'.

The difference is probably due to poverty. Relatively generous Swedish welfare benefits mean that only 6.8 per cent of their children live in families with less than half the average income. In Britain, on the other hand, the Child Poverty Action Group finds that one-third of all children are being raised in households living on or below the poverty line. If Swedish lone-parent families are not a breeding ground for social problems this, suggests Giddens, 'might be because, in societies such as the UK or the US, it is poverty rather than the family which is the true origin of . . . criminality and violence' (1997: 155).

If lone-parent families are not responsible for social problems, nor do rising divorce rates necessarily indicate that marriage is failing. The proportion of people who have been married at some point is actually *higher* than it was in the past, and most people who divorce will go on to remarry. Moreover the majority of births out of wedlock are better described as births *before* wedlock, since the majority are to parents who subsequently decide to marry (Abercrombie *et al.* 1994). Many social scientists suggest that people's willingness to end marriages indicates not that they are disillusioned with married life but that they have higher expectation of it than earlier generations, and are willing to make changes to achieve a *better* marriage (albeit with a new partner).

This is not to deny there have been important challenges to the nuclear family. Some have arisen from individuals and groups adopting a conscious,

political position that regards the nuclear family as problematic and promotes alternatives. Some early socialist critiques developed as early as the
nineteenth century, whilst others, such as the lesbian and gay argument for
'families of choice' are more recent.

These alternatives to the nuclear family include the following.

- The Commune Movement, which grew out of nineteenth-century
  socialist thought and experienced a revival in the 1960s, proposed
  communal living as more conducive to well-being than the narrow
  nuclear family. Groups of people pooled resources to purchase large
  rural houses with enough land to grow food or squatted in large town
  houses. The values of the Commune Movement incorporated concern
  for environmental issues and the redistribution of wealth, and some
  communes still exist.
- The Israeli kibbutz movement, which set up large communal farming
  communities as part of the 'greening of the desert', took place in the
  early days of the State of Israel. Children were cared for in communal
  nurseries and were seen as the responsibility of all.
- The women's movement had criticised the developing nuclear family
  as early as 1762, when Sarah Scott published *Millenium Hall*, describing
  a feminist communal household. Subsequently, 'second wave' feminists
  were responsible for exposing the darker side of the family by bringing
  to light issues such as domestic violence, marital rape and child sex
  abuse. Some experimented with communal living. However, mainstream
  feminists were more likely to demand *changes* in the family than its
  abolition.
- The anti-psychiatry movement of the 1960s, led by R.D. Laing, identified
  the nuclear family as an emotionally and psychologically destructive
  pressure cooker and claimed that the contradictions and repressed
  conflicts within families were responsible for schizophrenia. This critique
  led to the establishment of 'therapeutic communities', many of which
  still operate today.

Lesbian and gay families

To these developments must be added the ideas of the contemporary
lesbian and gay liberation movement. It is, of course, a mistake to imagine that there is agreement amongst lesbians and gay men about family
life and family structures. Factors other than simple politics impact on the
relationships that lesbians and gay men may have with their families of
origin and with their own children. We might expect this to lead to a
complex and contradictory set of ideas about family life, and this is indeed
the case.

One significant issue is the commonly shared experience of family
rejection and the emotional pain that results (Trenchard and Warren
1984; Whitlock 1988; Trenchard 1989; Stonewall 1999). This group are
not alone in finding families a source of pain. Abercrombie and his

colleagues, writing about family life (1994: 270), warn against assuming it is inevitably protective:

> If we appear to be unable to do without families, then they must be beneficial for us. We cannot assume that. For many people their family life is positively harmful and, probably for the majority of people, their experiences with families bring a good deal of pain as well as pleasure.

Although painful family experiences are very common, they are especially so for lesbians and gay men. Often rejected by their families of origin, prohibited by law from forming their own recognised partnerships, too often disregarded when trying to insist on next-of-kin status for their life partners, regarded as unfit to adopt or foster and constantly at risk of having their children taking away from them (Kaufmann and Lincoln 1991; Griffin and Mulholland 1997; Stacey 1997), this is perhaps the social group with most cause to claim that 'families bring a good deal of pain'. The profession of social work, which generally aims to protect and support family life, has regularly been instrumental in the destruction of lesbian or gay families (Cossis Brown 1992).

Gay dads, lesbian mums

Because of the very real risks faced by lesbian and gay parents it is difficult to establish exactly how many there are and estimates vary widely. In the United States, it is thought that there are between 1 million and 5 million lesbian mothers and between 1 million and 3 million gay fathers, and that an estimated 6–14 million children have a lesbian or gay parent (Singer and Deschamps 1994). Richardson's research into childrearing leads to an equally tentative conclusion. She writes that, 'In Britain, one in four children are now born to women who are not married, just over half of whom are living with a man. The other half includes lesbians, celibate and single heterosexual women' (Richardson 1993: 77). In other words, as many as one in eight children born in Britain *might* have a lesbian mother, but there is no way of knowing. Given that the majority of women who adopt a lesbian identity do so after living part of their adult lives as heterosexuals (Whisman 1996), it is likely that a significant proportion of the group described as 'lesbian mothers' became lesbians *after* becoming mothers.

However difficult it is to come to any accurate figures, it is clear that a substantial number of children are being reared in lesbian households and that a smaller (although still significant) number have at least regular contact with a gay father. Although attitudes are changing, these families still have to struggle against generally held prejudice; 'In 1987', according to Weeks (1991: 139), a British social attitudes survey revealed that '86 per cent would forbid lesbians adopting children, while an overwhelming 93 per cent would prevent gay men'. More recent local studies reveal that such families face problems with bullying at schools, lack of support from teachers and GPs, and hostility from neighbours and extended family members (Wilton and Hall 1998; Mugglestone 1999; Wilton 1999b).

They also have to contend with discriminatory laws; in the US no less than 11 states have rules that 'lesbians and gay men, on the basis of their sexual orientation, are unfit to receive custody of their children' (Singer and Deschamps 1994: 36), whilst in Britain the 1990 Human Fertilization and Embryology Bill contains a clause that effectively prohibits clinics providing fertility treatment to lesbians (Smith 1994). Richardson (1993: 77) concludes that, 'it is lesbian mothers in particular who face the greatest opposition to women openly choosing to have children outside marriage'.

In this context it is hardly surprising that lesbian and gay activists have put much time and effort into the fight to have their families recognised and to challenge the damaging myths about their being unfit to parent. Many studies have been carried out into the parenting practices of lesbians and gay men and their outcomes for the physical, intellectual and emotional well-being of the children. Such studies have proved conclusively that lesbian or gay parents are *not* more likely to rear homosexual children and that children from such families are at least as intelligent, healthy, secure and confident as their peers from heterosexual households. As Richardson points out (1993: 81), 'This ought not to matter. Lesbians should not have to prove that their children develop into "happy heterosexuals" in order to be considered fit to bring up children.' This is not a standard of proof that heterosexual parents have to meet, a point recognised in the popular T shirt slogan 'It takes two heterosexuals to make one homosexual'.

Indeed, Diane Richardson has asked why researchers have failed to explore the potentially *beneficial* consequences for children, pointing out for example that 'The evidence is that children, especially girls, being brought up in a lesbian household are at far less risk of sexual abuse than children raised in a household with a male parent present' (Richardson 1993: 81). Some researchers have found that 'lesbian mothers are actually more child-oriented than heterosexual mothers and that lesbian mothers are more concerned about the long-range development of their children' (Andersen 1988: 163). Such unbiased research as does exist offers an extremely positive account of the skills of lesbian and gay parents (Saffron 1994; Dunne 1998). Indeed, there was a brief press furore in the summer of 1999 when one major research project at the prestigious London School of Economics concluded that, in some respects, there may be advantages to a child in having lesbian parents (Dunne 1999).

We are family

While one section of the lesbian and gay community has been fighting for respect and legal recognition of their partnerships and parenting, another has been engaged in redefining 'family' in ways that more directly reject the heterosexual nuclear norm. In her major study of lesbian and gay kinship networks in the Bay area of San Francisco, Kath Weston found that entirely new models of family were being formed, incorporating lovers, ex-lovers, friends, children and blood kin in a variety of combinations. She identified an innovative approach at work, premised on the notion of 'family of choice', and introducing ideas of agency normally absent from family relationships. The old saying 'You can choose your friends but you can't choose your family' is being challenged by this large and disparate community, many of whom have experienced family rejection at first hand. Even for those whose blood family does not openly reject them, there may be a painful disruption of previously close ties, as described by one of Weston's interviewees:

> my family ties, before coming out, there was a lot of closeness. I could share stuff with my sisters. You used to talk all your deep dark secrets. You can't any more 'cause they think you're weird.
>
> (Weston 1998: 397)

The communities studied by Weston responded by creating new forms of family. She concludes (1998: 408) that:

> the possibility of being rejected by blood relatives for a lesbian or gay identity shaped the specific meanings carried by 'family' in gay contexts, undermining the permanence culturally attributed to blood ties while highlighting categories of choice and love . . . Most understood gay families to be customized, individual creations that need not deny conflict or difference.

Of course much sadness and pain accompanies lesbians and gay men as they try to develop alternative family bonds (Hargaden and Llewellin 1996), and it is important neither to underestimate the misery that may result, nor to romanticise the families of choice which can develop. Many of Weston's interviewees 'alluded to the difficulty *and excitement* of constructing kinship in the *absence* of what they called "models"' (1998: 397, first emphasis mine, second in original). However, they were living in a uniquely supportive environment.

More than a quarter of the population of San Francisco (>27.6 per cent) is known to be lesbian or gay (Singer and Deschamps 1994: 31), and the Bay area surveyed by Weston is a 'gay ghetto' with a very high concentration of gay households. Thus, lesbian and gay social networks are very strong, the services available locally are extremely supportive and there is less likelihood of meeting open hostility on a daily basis. This is a relatively privileged subcultural group, which therefore has more freedom and resources to devote to developing families of choice. It is likely to be more difficult for lesbians and gay men elsewhere to achieve this degree of creativity in their domestic lives. Nevertheless, the undoubted achievements of this small community offer exciting pointers to all those, whether gay or straight, who are seeking alternatives to the narrow 'cereal packet' norm.

Conclusion

This chapter has shown that 'family' is not a fixed, monolithic concept, nor is any particular family structure more natural, instinctive or benign than any other. An outline of the social history of the nuclear family demonstrates that a variety of family forms has alway existed, changing in response to shifting cultural, geopolitical, social and economic circumstances.

Sociologists agree that, in complex industrial societies, familial ideology is an intrinsic element in the policing of sexualities and of gender roles. Where the economic foundations of the nation state depend on a heterosexual division of labour, lesbian and gay families are extremely vulnerable to social exclusion and to being made scapegoats, along with other non-nuclear families, as a threat to family values and hence the state. Some scholars find the concept 'heteronormativity' useful to describe this complex socio-political process (see essays in Abelove *et al.* 1993; Siedman 1996; Lancaster and di Leonardo 1997).

The consequences of this situation pose a problem for health and social care (HSC), since it is difficult, and may be counter-productive, to impose a normative model of the family across an entire society. Those working in social care and, less directly, health care, are engaged in forms of professional intervention that privilege certain family forms over others. Historically, social services interventions have often contributed to the destruction of non-traditional families.

The organisational structures by which health and social care is delivered assume a heterosexual nuclear family norm, and hence, despite increasing recognition of the diversity of family forms, may contribute to heteronormativity. Sometimes, indeed, the reinforcement of heteronormative ideology is quite deliberate. When issues such as the reproductive rights of lesbians have been the subject of public debate we have seen that some HSC professionals – such as doctors and directors of social services – have gone on record to describe such developments as unnatural, undesirable or threatening to social stability.

In terms of individual practice, both ethics and professional reflexivity demand that those working in health and social care retain a critical awareness that ideas of the family are socio-political rather than natural, and that dominant norms tend to reflect the values of the most powerful groups in society. The struggle to balance the needs of patients and clients against the requirements of statutory authority has always been one of the most demanding aspects of a career in health or social care, and the contentious question of what a 'good family' looks like is a particularly immediate aspect of that struggle.

exercise

Read the following brief extract from an article published in 1945 in the *Journal of Personality.*

> Homosexuality is to a very large extent an acquired abnormality and propagates itself as a morally contagious disease. It tends to build up a society with even a kind of language of its own, and certainly with practices foreign to those of normal society. It tends to bring about more and more unfruitful unions that withdraw men and women from normal family life, the development of homes, and the procreation of children. The growth of a homosexual society in any country is a menace, more or less serious, to the welfare of the state.

Working either independently or in small groups, discuss the following points:

1 How many negative words or phrases are used in association with homosexuality? How many are positive or neutral? How is 'homosexuality' constructed by such language?

2 What do you make of the phrase 'practices foreign to normal society'? What practices do you think might be meant by this? What do you think of the implied contrast between the words 'foreign' and 'normal'?

3 To what extent does this extract medicalise homosexuality? What other research traditions are drawn on?

4 The extract clearly confirms a particular construct of homosexuality, but there is also a construct of heterosexuality perceptible. Identify the elements of this construct of heterosexuality and discuss them.

5 What do you suggest might be the possible *psychological* and *social* consequences for lesbians and gay men produced by articles such as this? What might be the consequences for heterosexuals?

6 Compare this extract with some of the more recent statements reported in this chapter. To what extent have attitudes changed since 1945?

Further reading

Dunne, G.A. (1997) *Lesbian Lifestyles: Women's Work and the Politics of Sexuality.* London: Macmillan.

Giddens, A. (1992) *The Transformation of Intimacy: Sexuality, Love and Eroticism in Modern Societies.* Cambridge: Polity.

Hague, G. and Malos, E. (1993) *Domestic Violence: Action for Change.* Cheltenham: New Clarion.

Richardson, D. (1993) *Women, Motherhood and Childrearing*. London: Macmillan.

Saffron, L. (1996) *What about the Children? Sons and Daughters of Lesbian and Gay Parents Speak about their Lives*. London: Cassell.

Sutcliffe, L. (1995) *There Must be 50 Ways to Tell Your Mother*. London: Cassell.

Weeks, J. (1991) *Against Nature: Essays on History, Sexuality and Identity*. London: Rivers Oram.

9 sexuality and public policy

Introduction

This chapter discusses the relationship between sexuality and citizenship, and explores the implications of this for the provision of public services. It outlines the restricted access that lesbians and gay men have to services which most heterosexuals take for granted, and examines some explanations for this state of affairs, concluding with an assessment of the role of the health and social care professions.

What is social policy?

A widely accepted, but fairly narrow, definition of social policy itself is that it consists of, 'the development and operation of state welfare policies and practices'. Similarly, the academic discipline known as 'social policy' is characterised by critical attempts to understand and/or theorise such policies and practices and their development (Williams 1989: 3). However, some areas of formally organised social life, such as the provision of local authority libraries and sports centres or the management of police forces, do not fit easily into the category of welfare as it is generally understood. It is therefore probably more useful to think of social policy as having to do with all services funded from the public purse, including those services that make up the 'welfare state' (such as health, social security and housing), but not limited to them.

The welfare state was established by the first Labour Government just as the Second World War came to an end. Its principles were outlined in the Beveridge Report of 1942, and its intention was to lay the foundations for a land fit for heroes. None of the problems identified by Beveridge have been eliminated from contemporary society. Nevertheless, the provisions of the welfare state were truly revolutionary, and the difference that they made to the lives of ordinary people was immense (H. Jones 1994).

All political interventions grow out of contemporary social circumstances and reflect perceptions of the time, and the foundation of the welfare state was no exception. In particular, it reflected key assumptions about gender and sexuality. As feminist critics have pointed out (Doyal with Pennell 1979; Maclean and Groves 1991), it was based on a very specific gendered division of labour, and on the unquestioned assumption that this was natural and permanent.

The architects of the welfare state assumed that full employment would be the norm, that men and women would marry and raise children in a nuclear family unit, that men would be the heads of household and would earn enough to support their families (the so-called 'family wage'), and that women would stay at home to look after the house, feed and care for the male bread-winner and his children, and provide any care which was needed by sick, disabled and elderly family members (Doyal with Pennell 1979; Williams 1989). In other words, the success of the welfare state depended on the unpaid labour of women at every stage in their adult life, and on adult men being employed continuously until retirement age.

From what we have learned already, it is not difficult to see that the implementation of such policies would act as a powerful reinforcement to specific ideas about gender-appropriate behaviour. Moreover, we might suspect that any infrastructure that depended on maintaining specific gender roles would prove vulnerable, over time, to changes in this area of social life.

Ironically, of course, the social trends which would bring such huge pressure to bear on state-funded services were already well advanced by the 1940s. Social transformations, such as the entry of women into higher education and into new segments of the labour market, rising rates of divorce and changing attitudes to non-procreative sexual activity were all gathering speed by this time. Hence the notion of a fixed and stable heterosexual family structure was not a reliable foundation for the creation of a 'welfare state'.

Many of the social changes that have made these services so difficult to sustain have been in the area of gender and sexuality. The implications of gender have been well theorised within the discipline of social policy. Sexuality, however, remains almost completely neglected. A small number of analysts are starting to discuss sexuality in the context of political theory (see, for example, Smith 1994; Richardson 1998), but most books on social policy fail to refer to the issue at all (see, for example, Williams 1989; Maclean and Groves 1991; George and Miller 1994; L. Jones 1994). Yet sexuality is a key issue in debates around citizenship, social inclusion and exclusion and access to public services, including health and social care.

Many feminists would argue that women remain 'invisible' within the welfare state (see, for example, Maclean and Groves 1991). It is therefore to be expected that lesbians and gay men will each have very different experiences of public service provision. In order fully to understand the relationship between individuals and public services such as health care or the police, we must therefore consider both gender *and* sexuality. Any discussion of the problems of single mothers, for example, will be greatly enriched by identifying the different ways in which lone parenting is experienced by lesbian and non-lesbian mothers.

Citizenship, rights and duties

To be the citizen of a nation state is to have certain rights and responsibilities – 'civil rights' – some of which are enshrined in law. Even at this very basic level, gender and sexuality have an important effect. Citizenship is not a gender-neutral concept. The 'typical' citizen is almost always assumed to be male. Dunn points out that: 'the duty to give life, should it be necessary to do so, in order to maintain or generate a political order, is one of the central duties of citizenship' (Dunn 1980, cited in Pateman 1992: 23). This duty, of course, generally (until recently, exclusively) applies to men.

On this count, gay men are immediately excluded from citizenship in countries (such as the US at the time of writing) which prohibit them from serving in the military. This is why lesbian and gay groups are campaigning for the right to serve in the military; not because they are an unusually militaristic group but because denial of this right effectively excludes them from full citizenship status.

Women, it has been argued, are granted a limited form of citizenship relative to that of men. Women traditionally achieve what citizenship rights they are allowed by exercising their reproductive capacity in the interests of the state. As Pateman summarises:

Motherhood, as feminists have understood for a very long time, exists as a central mechanism through which women have been incorporated into the modern political order. Women's service and duty to the state have largely been seen in terms of motherhood, and . . . women's duty is connected to men's service to the state as workers and soldiers.

(Pateman 1992: 19)

The historical origins of the British welfare state are, then, closely bound up with warfare, and most key elements of welfare legislation concern either the health of women and children or the health of men as workers. Innovations such as the school meals service were prompted in large part by the very poor health of recruits to the Boer War and the First and Second World Wars (Doyal with Pennell 1979; H. Jones 1994).

If, as it appears, female citizenship is so closely linked to women's reproductive success, this raises interesting questions about the ways in which British politicians have intervened to make it impossible for lesbians to become mothers. At various times since 1980, Parliament has considered legislation to prevent clinics providing fertility treatment to lesbians (indeed, to all single women); to make it illegal for local authorities to place children with lesbian or gay foster parents; to prevent lesbians adopting children; and to prevent discussion about lesbian and gay families from taking place in schools (Smith 1994). Parliamentary records and the wording of both proposed and enacted legislation – such as the contentious reference to lesbian and gay families as 'pretended' in Section 28 of the 1988 Local Government Act – make it clear that lesbians have not been regarded as 'real' mothers at all (Colvin and Hawksley 1989).

Marriage

Lesbian and gay activists have long protested the fact that a married relationship is universally promoted by the state and its institutions as being the best environment in which to rear a child whilst at the same time, lesbians and gay men are prevented by law from marrying (Stonewall 1999). Some argue that this is because marriage must be reserved for those couples who are biologically able to produce children. However, this argument simply does not hold up. There have, for example, been no moves to ban women past childbearing age from marrying, nor to declare null and void the marriages of those who choose not to have children. Such inconsistencies seem to support Richardson's finding that 'claims to citizenship status, at least in the West, are closely associated with the institutionalisation of heterosexual as well as male privilege' (Richardson 1998: 88).

The vexed question of gay marriage demonstrates that the relationship between the British state and its lesbian and gay citizens is unique insofar as the state actively intervenes to *prevent* them both fulfilling the obligations and reponsibilities of citizenship and benefiting from its privileges. Since this group pay exactly the same rates of tax, national insurance and community charge as their heterosexual peers, this is unjust (Trades Unionists against Section 28 1989; Tatchell 1992).

Marriage is also an important aspect of the economic inequalities faced by lesbians and gay men. Although some sociologists suggest that marriage is in the process of becoming redundant (Giddens 1994), it nevertheless carries significant economic advantages. Pensions and insurance schemes, whether statutory or private, recognise the claims of a spouse as legitimate, and as such the surviving member of a married couple has specific entitlements on the death of their spouse. State benefits include the payment of a widow's pension and tax benefits associated with marriage.

These statutory arrangements are grossly inadequate; widowhood or divorce may carry particularly severe financial penalties for women (Kember 1997); but they do provide some protection, however minimal, which is unavailable to same-sex partners. Of course, certain elements of the economic privileges of marriage are also withheld from cohabiting heterosexual couples but, unless circumstances are exceptional, heterosexuals generally have the choice whether or not to marry.

The international context

In seeking to deny lesbians and gay men the rights and responsibilities of full citizenship, Britain is no different from the United States and from most other nation states in the global community. Partial exceptions are to be found in some countries such as Brazil, South Africa, Canada or parts of Scandinavia. In Denmark and Sweden, for example, same-sex couples may register their partnerships in a ceremony that gives some (but not all) of the benefits of marriage. Significantly, however, this partnership legislation stated that such couples are not allowed to adopt children (Bech 1992). More hopeful signs include the decision to incorporate lesbian and gay rights in the constitution of post-apartheid South Africa, and recognition of the civil rights of this group is slowly growing in countries such as Canada, Eire and Australia.

It is difficult to explain the continued withholding of civil rights in Britain and elsewhere, since other 'unpopular' groups – including criminals, alcoholics, drug abusers and even murderers – do not have their civil status compromised in this way. Indeed, contemporary democracies are founded on important beliefs about the civil and human rights of individuals, and about the requirement to accord such rights respect and, where necessary, protection.

Yet, as Richardson finds in her analysis of citizenship (1998: 92):

it would seem that very often the role of sexuality in the construction of concepts of nationality is not merely linked to heterosexuality, but to a form of heterosexuality that is to varying extents anti-lesbian as well as anti-gay.

Why is it the case that people who choose members of their own sex to be their intimate, sexual and domestic partners are routinely denied basic rights, including in some circumstances and in some places the right to life itself? And why is this situation so widely perceived as right and proper? The next section looks at how scholars have interpreted this situation.

Bureaucracies and homosexuality

Until relatively recently, the stigma against homosexuality in Euro-American societies was so deeply rooted that it was not thought necessary to explain why being homosexual disqualified one from basic human and civil rights. Historically there have been many attempts to justify the situation. Justifications have been based on religious concepts of sin, medical notions of sickness or political assertions that homosexuals represent a risk to national security, but justifications are not explanations.

Any attempt to explain the political exclusion of lesbians and gay men must begin by analysing the socio-political nature of that which excludes them. Such an approach requires us to study the apparatus and ideology of the state as *producing* the problem rather than simply responding to an existing situation.

Some social scientists suggest that every 'in group' needs an 'out group' in order to define itself and that homosexuals just happen to form one of the unfortunate 'out groups'. While this may describe the process of social exclusion and offer a generalised rationale for its continuance, it does little to explain why particular groups are singled out. Others have argued that complex industrial societies are organised around highly formalised hierarchies, and that social organisation may be subverted by the existence of a gay subculture, which enables men to form intimate relationships across such hierarchies:

> Homosexual desire links men who otherwise would not be linked: homosexuals are men who are brought together not by money and property interest but by sex ... Such groupings are not structured according to the 'proper' orders of society, such as nation, class and profession.
>
> (Shepherd 1989: 215)

Still others suggest that the political exclusion of lesbians and gay men is bound up with old notions of homosexuality as a gender inversion, since the nation state is an institution closely linked to male power and since (as we have seen) it depends on the heterosexual nuclear family to function smoothly (Faderman 1985; Wittig 1992).

There is some evidence for this in the public statements of right-wing British politicians. Margaret Thatcher, for example, once famously insisted that 'A nation of free people will only continue to be great if family life continues and the structure of that nation is a family one' (cited in Sanderson 1995: 229). A very similar position was taken by Ian Paisley when he spoke out against proposed legislation to bring the age of consent for gay men into line with that for heterosexuals and lesbians: 'This country must realize that the unit of society, and the cement that holds it together, is the family . . . The normal sex act within the marriage vow, bringing together male and female and producing offspring, is the happy way; it is the divine way . . .' (cited in Saraga 1998: 184). Public statements such as these lend credence to the theory that the state discriminates against its lesbian and gay citizens because same-sex partnerships cannot biologically produce children. Yet this cannot be a full explanation for, as we have seen, much time and energy is expended in order to *prevent the development* of lesbian and gay family units with children.

Another explanation focuses on the perceived need to maintain popular support for the very abstract ideas that go to make up the existence of a nation state. This theory is supported by an analysis of circumstances in which homosexuality has been linked to treachery or treason. Simon Shepherd (1989: 223) has researched social attitudes in Nazi Germany, the McCarthy era in America and Cold-War Britain and comments, 'Homosexual treachery stories tend to surface in conditions of national "pride" and reconstruction.' He concludes that such stories 'may be useful to a state that is occupied in constructing a sense of national community', and goes on to suggest that certain forms of government may in fact *need* the fantasy figure of the treacherous homosexual in order to maintain their authority:

> by agreeing to the fixed rules of class and gender status, one can be assured of one's secure place in the 'national community' . . . Stories of queer treachery, comprising as they do allegiances to class, gender system and race, are powerful devices for maintaining people's consent to the fabricated idea of nation.
>
> (Shepherd 1989: 225)

There are powerful arguments in support of this interpretation. However, it does not apply so neatly to lesbians. Nor can it easily explain why the same nation state may seem to shift from extreme oppression of its lesbian and gay citizens to a much more liberal and tolerant approach in a relatively short space of time.

Sociologist David Greenberg has used Weber's classical sociological concept of the ideal bureaucracy – 'ideal' in the sense of typical rather than 'best possible' – in an attempt to understand lesbian and gay political exclusion. One of the advantages of this approach is that it enables us to study this situation as just one of many forms of exclusion associated with bureaucratic societies and to assess the similarities and differences between them.

Bureaucracies, in the Weberian sense, are characterised by a segregation of official activities from the world of private life, by administration on the basis of general rules and regulations, and by impersonality. Bureaucratic governments depend on salaried officials to administer and enforce rules and regulations. One important consequence of this is that it is relatively simple to repress groups or activities. For example, someone who is disturbed by a neighbour's dog barking may lodge a formal complaint with the existing authorities, whose job it is to pursue the matter. This course of action carries much lower costs than face-to-face confrontation in terms of energy, time and personal risk, and provides regular work for those paid to intervene in such circumstances.

There are many positive elements to this aspect of bureaucracy. However, citizens in a bureaucratically organised state may pay a heavy price in the form of a greatly increased potential for social control and repression. This is why the 'faceless bureaurocrat' has become such a symbol of frustration and anxiety, for when repression becomes easy, it also becomes more likely:

> the existence of an enforcement bureaucracy removes obstacles to the repression of activities that are only mildly offensive to the general population . . . Since costs are distributed to all taxpayers, they are not excessively burdensome to any one person, and even those who are not particularly in favour of repression are unlikely to protest.
>
> (Greenberg 1988: 435–436)

Greenberg's study found that bureaucratic institutions have historically been characterised by repressive attitudes to homosexuality. He finds this to be true of institutions as varied as the Spanish Inquisition, Revolutionary Cuba, the Stalinist Soviet Union, the US military and Nazi Germany; all of which were/are highly bureaucratic and authoritarian. The ease with which bureaucratic regimes are able to repress behaviours which they deem unacceptable does explain why discrimination against lesbians and gay men generally goes unchallenged even by those who do not consider themselves homophobic. However, it does not explain *why* homosexuality is unacceptable to bureaucratic societies, nor why sexuality *per se* figures so largely in bureaucratic social control. Where repression is facilitated by bureaucracy, why are lesbians and gay men repressed rather than, say, vegetarians?

The usefulness of Greenberg's work lies in his exploration of these questions. Many sociologists have studied the 'bureaucratic personality' that is required by bureaucratic organisations and which is produced by socialisation and education; Greenberg tentatively identifies this as an important element in the exclusion of homosexuals:

> Because the formation of the bureaucratic personality in men entails the suppression of affective emotional responses towards males, men will tend to experience anxiety in the presence of emotional intimacy or sexual contact between men . . . It is this anxiety, I contend, that lies behind irrational anger towards male homosexuality.
>
> (Greenberg 1988: 447)

This suggestion is useful because it offers a plausible explanation, not simply for homophobic violence but for some important differences between the experiences of lesbians and of gay men. Greenberg elaborates further, discussing the very high degrees of homophobic exclusion present in 'total' institutions such as the military, and the role of the police in the harassment and entrapment of gay men.

However, the state and the provision of public services within the statutory sector are extremely complex, and the forms that exclusion may take are no less complex. It is unlikely that any single theory will be completely adequate to the task of fully explaining the relationship between sexuality and political exclusion across all societies, but Greenberg's work remains the most useful to date.

Sexual orientation and access to public services

Whatever the explanations for their political exclusion, research indicates that lesbians and gay men in Britain are discriminated against in all areas of service provision (Galloway 1983; Kaufmann and Lincoln 1991; Sheffield Health 1996; Wilton 1999b). Tatchell finds, for example (1992: 237), that 'about twenty different points of law, either explicitly or by omission, discriminate against the lesbian and gay community'.

It is noteworthy that even critical accounts of public service provision very seldom recognise lesbians and/or gay men as a service user group. Nor do they make any attempt to account for sexuality as a significant social variable when discussing social policy. Even feminist researchers and writers, who might reasonably be expected to recognise the significance of sexuality in relation to gender, generally ignore the existence of lesbians (see, for example, Williams 1989; Maclean and Groves 1991; Pennell Initiative 1998). The heterosexism of this literature (Wilton 1993) makes it difficult for care professionals to get access to the specific information they need when developing appropriate services for this group. Relevant information is more likely to be found in the literature of lesbian and gay studies; a discipline unlikely to be familiar to most health and social care practitioners or students.

Paid employment

Although paid employment is not a public service in the generally accepted meaning of the word, policy issues affecting lesbian and gay employment may have important consequences for access to services. Employment status, for example, has a direct bearing on use of public services and entitlement to certain benefits.

At the time of writing there are moves afoot to provide legal protection for the employment rights of lesbians and gay men in the UK (Stonewall 1999). Until this happens (and there remains fierce opposition in many quarters), it is still perfectly legal to fire an employee simply because of their sexual orientation. A Trades Union working party found that:

> There is no specific protection for lesbians and gay men against discrimination by employers . . .

> Courts and tribunals are biased towards employers and tradition-
> ally unsympathetic to lesbians and gay men.
> The laws on discrimination are inadequate and apply only to race
> and sex . . .
> Legal remedies are individual, not collective . . . employers are at
> liberty to ignore these judgements until challenged in the courts by
> another aggrieved individual.
>
> (Trades Unionists Against Section 28 1989: 7)

In the face of this lack of legislative protection, it is crucial that workplace
equal opportunities policies specifically include sexual orientation, since
such policies currently offer the *only* protection available to workers.
Moreover, the lack of legislation to protect lesbian and gay employment
rights contributes to a general assumption that such discrimination is
acceptable.

Working in such a vulnerable situation has been found to compromise
the health and well-being of lesbians and gay men (Sheffield Health
1996; Wilton 1997b; Mugglestone 1999). They face an inevitably stressful
choice between hiding an important part of themselves or risking the
harassment of colleagues and even dismissal. Not surprisingly, the employment opportunities open to this group have long been severely restricted
in consequence, with large numbers choosing to work below their abilities
or qualifications in low-paid jobs, often in the service sector (Davies 1996).

There are, of course, occupations that offer some protection against discrimination and a few traditionally hostile employers, such as the Police,
are beginning to recognise the unacceptable costs of disciminatory employment practices which exclude large numbers of potentially talented
employees. Nevertheless, the relative safety of a few working environments
should not be taken as the norm. For example, whilst institutions in
higher education are slowly incorporating sexuality into their equal opportunities statements, this is emphatically *not* the case for education generally,
and school teaching remains one area where the harassment of lesbian or
gay employees can quickly turn into a witchhunt, as the media hounding
of primary headteacher Jane Brown in 1994 illustrates only too clearly
(Sanderson 1995).

Not only do lesbian and gay employees lack the employment rights
that heterosexual employees take for granted, they also miss out on
many work-related benefits. The protection that pension schemes offer to
surviving partners in the case of death or severe injury only apply to
married partners. Other work-related perks, such as discounts on company
products or travel privileges may also be regarded as for heterosexual
partners, and so far the courts have upheld the legality of this exclusion-
ary practice, since there are no existing laws to prohibit it. Unions such as
the National Association of Local Government Employees (NALGO) and
the National Association of Teachers in Further and Higher Education
(NATFHE) are increasingly concerned that lesbian and gay employees are
financially subsidising their heterosexual colleagues by considerable sums
via such discriminatory practices.

The lack of employment rights for lesbians and gay men, coupled with the inequitable distribution of the financial rewards of paid work, put this group in a unique position with regard to public services. This is seldom recognised by policy makers, nor by academics or researchers. This lack of awareness is due in part to ingrained heterosexism, but may also reflect assumptions about the lifestyles of more privileged, and hence more socially visible, lesbians and gay men. Two educated, professional gay men living together in a stable couple relationship may well be economically privileged; being less likely to have children than their non-gay peers both will have an uninterrupted career pattern and their disposable income will not be reduced by child-rearing expenses.

However, this degree of economic privilege is far from being the norm. It is not shared by lesbian couples, whose access to the labour market is more restricted by sexism, discrimination and responsibility for bringing up children (Dunne 1997). Nor is it shared by the less visible majority of gay men, those whose age, class or ethnic background, whose lack of educational advantage or marketable skills mean that they are confined to less secure and less well paid work. Though further research is needed, there can be little doubt that the employment insecurity, which is such a major factor in the lives of most lesbians and gay men, has far-reaching consequences for their health and well-being.

Housing

Housing provision in Britain changed dramatically as a result of the introduction of a 'right to buy' policy, whereby those in council owned housing were enabled to buy their homes. The amount of publicly owned housing available at low rent to those in need decreased dramatically in consequence. At the same time, legal protection for tenants of private landlords was weakened and private rents rose above the reach of many. The withdrawal of benefit entitlement to young adults also made it impossible for this group to afford independent housing. The results have been a large increase in mortgage arrears and repossessions by mortgage lenders, a chronic shortage of local authority housing for those most in need, an increase in those living in bed and breakfast accommodation, hostels and other forms of crisis accommodation, and a dramatically visible increase in the numbers of homeless people living on the street (Graham 1997; Millar 1997).

Homelessness charities and housing organisations are slowly beginning to recognise that sexual orientation has profound consequences for access to housing (Greater London Council 1985; Cookson 1988; Steel 1998). Indeed, London Lesbian and Gay Switchboard receives more calls each year for advice on housing problems than any other organisation in the country, including specialist housing agencies. The issues are simple. First, lesbians and gay men may be *more* likely to face homelessness. Young people are frequently thrown out of the family home when their parents become aware of their homosexuality, or they may be forced to leave by intolerable levels of hostility, violence, abuse or attempts to 'cure' them (Steel 1998).

Adults, too, may face specific problems. Insurance companies often have provisos relating to AIDS, which make it difficult for gay men to get life insurance in order to take out a mortgage, and the low-paid, insecure jobs on which many lesbians and gay men are dependent are often not enough to support a mortgage application or to fund the rents and deposits required by private landlords. One survey revealed that 40 per cent of those needing housing advice from London Lesbian and Gay Switchboard had been made homeless as a direct consequence of their sexuality (Trenchard and Warren 1984)

Traditional public housing policies are devised to support the stereotypical nuclear family. In a time when family structure is rapidly changing, such traditional policies have failed to keep up with the realities of people's requirements, and there are specific failures with regard to lesbians and gay men. In the area of youth homelessness, for example, one large-scale survey found that:

> Young gay men and lesbians are reluctant to use traditional homeless provision such as hostels due to the prevalence of anti-gay attitudes. They may move from place to place until they find somewhere relatively sympathetic.
>
> (Evans 1996: 14)

Lesbians with children are often dealt with as single parents by housing agencies, and there is plentiful evidence that single parents are discrimated against in local authority housing provision, often being allocated hard-to-let units (Wilton 1995). Few local authorities recognise same-sex couples' tenancy rights so, in the event of one dying, the surviving partner may face eviction following closely on the heels of bereavement. This may have a particularly devastating effect on older lesbians and gay men, who are also unlikely to have their needs recognised if they move into residential care.

Single, childless adults have little or no claim on welfare services and are pretty much left to fend for themselves. Since many benefits are contributions-linked, and since women's earning power remains less than men's, the safety net of benefits and pensions fails many never-married women. This is another under-researched area, but it is probable that many elderly lesbians, unable to claim widow's pensions or to benefit from the other financial entitlements that marriage brings, are living in poverty (Wilton 1995). This being the case, it is especially troubling that researchers continue to ignore the existence of this especially vulnerable group (see, for example, Pennell Initiative 1998).

The lesbian and gay community has fought for recognition for such problems. However, far more attention has been directed towards the plight of homelessness among lesbian and gay youth than among the elders of the community, and there is little understanding of the housing problems faced by lesbian mothers (Wilton 1995; Steel 1998). There are a few specialist agencies, which have grown out of lesbian and gay activism;

these include the Stonewall Housing action group, which offers supported housing to homeless 15–16-year-old lesbians and gay men in London and the Albert Kennedy Trust in London and Manchester, which provides services for those under 20 years of age. However, such specialist provision as exists is often dependent on community fund-raising, and is able to deal only with the tip of the iceberg of lesbian and gay homelessness.

The education service and youth work

Homophobia has a particularly nasty face when the question of children and young people is raised. Despite the uncontested fact that 95 per cent of child sex abuse is perpetrated by heterosexuals (Rochlin 1992), the assumption that homosexuals are child molesters remains deeply embedded. That it should retain its firm hold on the public imagination, despite all evidence to the contrary, is hardly surprising since the groups who campaign against lesbian and gay civil rights routinely declare that their chief aim is to *protect children* from homosexual perverts.

The risk to children is said to be twofold: first, that lesbian or gay adults might sexually abuse them and second, that they might be 'converted' or 'recruited' to a homosexual identity themselves. 'There is, of course,' write psychotherapists Hargaden and Llewellin (1996: 120), 'no evidence to support these prejudices . . . Nevertheless, they are frequently part of the cultural belief system by which we have [all] been influenced.'

This cultural belief system is readily manipulated. In the US, for example, Anita Bryant succeeded in defeating a proposed measure in the State of Oregon that would have outlawed discrimination on the grounds of sexual orientation. She called her campaign 'Save Our Children' and repeatedly insisted that 'homosexuals cannot reproduce, so they have to recruit our children'. As Cruikshank (1992: 15) comments, 'Bryant and her followers successfully persuaded voters to equate anti-discriminatory laws with child molesting, gay "recruiting", prostitution, threats to the family, and a national gay conspiracy.' Although the religious right is less influential in Britain than in the US, its influence is growing (Powell 1998).

The many parliamentary debates on various aspects of homosexuality may be read in Hansard, the official Parliamentary record. Such records are notable for the extraordinarily negative attitudes towards homosexuality shown by all sides. For example, when the ground-breaking Sexual Offences Bill (which partially decriminalised sex between men) was debated in the House, those speaking in support were clearly just as horrified by homosexuality as those opposing:

> I believe that the worst failure of the present law is the preoccupation with punishment of homosexuals which leads to the community not taking the preventative action which might possibly save a little boy from the terrible fate of growing up a homosexual . . . there are dangers to a boy if an over-possessive mother ties him to her with a silver cord, so that the boy, enveloped in a feminine aura, is never able to

break out and assert his masculine independence . . . A lad without a father . . . is sometimes left with a curse . . . of a male body encasing a feminine soul.

(Leo Abse, promoter of the Bill, 5 July 1966)

I sincerely believe that if the Bill is passed it will increase homosexual practices and not reduce them. It will not cleanse the national bloodstream; it will corrupt and poison it.

(Captain Elliot, opposing the Bill, 19 December 1966)

Nearly 30 years later, similar concerns were expressed by MPs debating equalising the age of consent for gay men:

it is neither natural nor normal to carry out homosexual activity. That is why there has to be protection for young boys. It is a different matter if they participate in that which is normal and natural, but if they are guided into activities that are neither normal nor natural, protection is required.

(Bill Walker, opposing)
(all three extracts cited in Saraga 1998: 177–184)

These extracts from Parliamentary debates are important, as they reveal the extent to which the myth of childhood induction into homosexuality permeates British society, and the anxiety to *protect* young men from anything that might result in their becoming homosexual.

There has not been the same degree of concern to protect young women, and it remains an interesting question why this is so. Lesbianism is routinely dismissed in the Parliamentary record of the twentieth century as fairly harmless (Smith 1992). The fear that young boys might be seduced into homosexuality is, in contrast, almost obsessive.

Although the question of identity formation remains contentious, there is no evidence of same-sex encounters in childhood or youth 'making' people gay. The few accounts where such encounters are described as positive make it very clear that the individuals in question were *already* gay at the time the encounter took place (Herdt 1989; Gonsiorek and Weinrich 1991; Porter and Weeks 1991; Sears 1991). It is also worth noting two other aspects of the 'gay seduction' argument. The first is that it is circular, proposing that homosexuality is bad sexuality – otherwise there would be no point in trying to prevent young men growing up gay – but arguing that it is bad *because* young men who encounter homosexuality may grow up gay. The second is that the assumption that gay men become that way because they were seduced as youngsters sits uneasily alongside the equally common belief that women may be driven into lesbianism as a result of sexual abuse by men.

Looked at critically, these common assumptions reveal something very strange indeed about our cultural notions of adult male sexuality. Although sexual encounters with adult men are held to be so pleasurable as to increase the likelihood of young men trying to repeat the experience (this is the implication of the gay seduction argument), young *women* who experience sexual encounters with adult men are commonly assumed to be so damaged by the event that they adopt a lesbian identity to avoid ever having this unpleasant experience again. In other words, it is thought *more pleasurable* for a man to have sex with another man than it is for a woman. Neither psychologists nor sociologists have yet developed a theoretical explanation for this anomaly.

The confused and misinformed notions that saturate official discourse on homosexuality have been particularly influential in education and youth work. This was most effectively demonstrated in the 'family values' campaign of the Thatcher administration (Sanders and Spraggs 1989; Kaufmann and Lincoln 1991; Weeks 1991; Smith 1992, 1994), which prioritised an explicit programme attacking lesbian and gay civil rights.

The tenor of this campaign may be judged by the words of Margaret Thatcher herself who, in her address to the Conservative Party Conference in 1987, complained that, 'Children who need to be taught to respect traditional values are being taught that they have an inalienable right to be gay' (Sanders and Spraggs 1989). There are two disturbing assumptions in this statement. The first is that 'traditional moral values' are the exclusive preserve of heterosexuals and the second is that individuals do not have the right to a self-determined sexuality. Thatcher's statement takes it as given that sexuality, far from being a private matter for individuals, is the proper business of the state.

With this in mind, the government of the time passed laws and issued directives in an attempt to protect young people from homosexuality *per se*. Section 28 of the 1988 Local Government Act was an attempt to prevent schools from teaching pupils about lesbian and gay lives, and government directives about sex education, such as Circular 11/87 from the Department of Education and Science, made it clear that there was an official requirement to promote sex within marriage as the only acceptable form of sexual activity (Department of Education and Science 1987; Aggleton *et al.* 1990).

A few local authorities did take seriously their responsibility to protect young lesbians and gay men in their care from abuse or assault, and developed equal opportunities policies to this end. Such policies were widely attacked. Tottenham Conservative Party, for example, publicly condemned the attempts of one such authority to provide support to their lesbian and gay young people as 'a greater threat to family life than Adolf Hitler' (Cooper 1989).

Adolescence is a trying time for many young people, and it does not take much imagination to realise that it is likely to be significantly more difficult for young lesbians and gay men. This assumption is borne out by research, both in the United States and in the UK, which shows that they are particularly likely to be bullied or assaulted, to be rejected by their parents and other family members, to be homeless, to have problems with alcohol and substance abuse and to attempt suicide (Trenchard and Warren 1984; Whitlock 1988; Herdt 1989; Epstein 1994).

It is especially significant that large numbers of young people are rejected by their families on account of their sexual orientation. This means that this particularly vulnerable group of young people are perhaps *more* in need of sympathetic, informed and aware adult support than their heterosexual peers. Yet, because the myth of homosexual seduction continues to influence policy makers, lesbian or gay adults who want to work with young people are viewed with deep suspicion. Many heterosexuals believe that homosexuality is in itself a proper reason for firing a teacher, youth worker or social worker. Indeed some states in the US have attempted to pass legislation forbidding state schools hiring lesbian or gay staff (Harvard Law Review 1989; Gomez *et al.* 1995). In the UK, the response of some local government officers to a national survey about this issue makes depressing reading:

> I would not, in normal circumstances, be prepared to condone the employment of homosexual men and women in posts in this department which carry a responsibility for the care of people and especially the care of children.
>
> (social services officer, Hampshire)

> Your audacity is beyond belief . . . to suggest that homosexuals should be allowed to work with vulnerable children is uppalling, I wonder would H. Sammuels employ a kleptomaniac . . . I can assure you that if it is brought to my knowledge that person with these tendencies are employed in the Social Services Department of the authority that I represent I shall do everything in my power to have them removed.
>
> (social services officer, West Yorkshire: spelling as in original)
>
> (both extracts from Dobson 1983: 47/51)

Lesbian and gay teachers and youth workers have worked hard to change this unhappy situation. Forming *ad hoc* professional support groups, such as the Gay Teachers' Group (GTG) and the National Organization of Lesbian and Gay Youth and Community Workers (NOLGYCW), and working with sympathetic professional bodies such as the National Organization for Work with Girls and Young Women (NOWGYW) and the British Youth Council (BYC), they have ensured that questions about sexuality remain on the agenda of those who work with young people and (importantly) of those responsible for their training. Attitudes are slowly shifting, and key national bodies such as Barnardos are starting to develop policies that recognise the existence and the particular needs of lesbian and gay youth. However, progress remains slow.

Guardians of the law: who is protected from whom?

One area of public policy where there have been important and much-needed changes in recent years is policing. Until the late 1990s there could be no doubt that most regional police forces were regarded as the enemy of local lesbian and gay communities. As one gay activist concluded:

No body is so resented by homosexuals as the police . . . Most gays feel threatened by the police. An employer, priest or doctor may make your life unpleasant. The police can put you behind bars.

(Galloway 1983: 102)

The belief that homosexuality was decriminalised in the wake of the Wolfenden Report is only partly true. The law recognises only the right of two consenting adults to have sex in private, and this may be interpreted with painstaking literalness by police and judiciary alike. It is, strictly speaking, illegal for two men to engage in any kind of sexual activity in any premises where there may be others present; in a hotel or club, during a private party, or in the bedroom of a house shared with others. It is also illegal for anyone to engage in any behaviour likely to cause a breach of the peace. This has been interpreted very widely; in some instances cases have been brought against individuals for holding hands, embracing, or kissing each other goodbye at train stations (Galloway 1983).

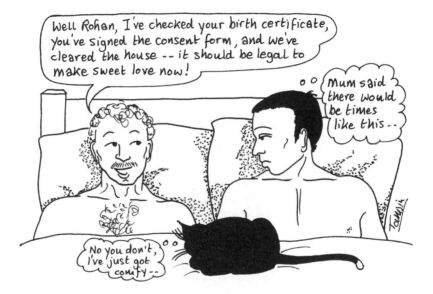

Evidence from civil rights groups make it clear that police officers have historically exploited whatever opportunity the law afforded them in order to harass the gay community. Pubs and clubs have been raided, 'pretty police' have hung about in public toilets trying to seduce men into making a pass at them, police have even raided private parties and arrested guests (Crane 1982; Galloway 1983; Kaufmann and Lincoln 1991; Porter and Weeks 1991).

More disturbing is the failure of the police to act in cases of gay-bashing. Indeed, there is evidence that officers may themselves be per-petrators, with gay men being extremely vulnerable to abuse and assault whilst in police custody (Galloway 1983; Connell 1987; Mason and Palmer 1997). Homophobic violence was such a common feature of police life that retired chief constable James Alderson suspected that there was something about being a policeman which encouraged it. 'I think,' he commented, 'there is a macho self-image about the police. I often wonder whether the police macho doesn't somehow feel itself threatened by homosexuality' (Galloway 1983: 103).

When gay men who have been the victims of violent assaults try to get police help, that help is all too often withheld. Recorded incidents suggest that gay bashing, in common with domestic violence and racist attacks, is either not taken seriously or is actively condoned by senior officers (Galloway 1983; Connell 1987; Mason and Palmer 1997). In one incident, 'one gay man who was attacked . . . had reason to doubt the peace-keeping role [of the police]. After staggering on the road in front of a police car he was himself arrested' (Deer 1980).

The troubled relationship between the gay community and the police was recognised by future Home Secretary Jack Straw in his foreword to a recent report on gay bashing:

> Today, although our society is thankfully more open and accepting of gay relationships, gay people are still disproportionately likely to be the victims of harassment and attack . . . the result is that lesbians and gay men adopt avoidance strategies of their own to guard against abuse, attacks may go unreported and criminals are often left unpunished. As one respondent put it: 'many people do not feel that the legal system and the police are there for them.'
>
> (Straw, in Mason and Palmer 1997)

The law on homosexuality is currently the subject of lively debate amongst lawyers and criminologists, for it is not clear who it protects and from what they are being protected. Most of the offences of which gay men are convicted are classic 'victimless crimes'. They involve consensual activities and damage nobody.

There are encouraging signs that some police forces are starting to recognise their failings and responsibilities in this area. Following the success of liaisons with women's groups, minority ethnic communities and others, lesbian and gay police liason groups now exist in 15 forces. Some police forces have begun recruiting lesbian and gay officers, and there is now a lesbian and gay police association. Mason and Palmer (1997: 84) found that, 'in the last five years, 41 out of 43 police forces have adopted new management policies that recognise the principle of equal treatment for lesbians and gay men'. The future of policing seems to offer some hope for optimism.

However, a word of caution is required. It has taken a very long time for racism to be accepted as a problem in policing. The inquiry into the death of Black teenager Stephen Lawrence, continuing unease about the frequency with which Black people die or are injured in police custody and many other questions make it clear that work on this issue is only just beginning. Change happens slowly and homophobia has a long history in the police. It was a policeman, James Anderton of the Greater

Manchester Force, who responded to the HIV pandemic with one of the most famously homophobic pronouncements of the time:

> Why do homosexuals continue sleeping with each other? Why do they still engage in sodomy and other obnoxious sexual practices knowing the dangers involved? We should ask them head on and challenge them to answer it. People at risk are swirling around in a cesspit of their own making.
>
> (Sanderson 1995: 207)

At the time that Anderton made this speech health officials were wringing their hands over the difficulties of getting stubborn *heterosexual* men to take responsibility for their behaviour, while heaping praise on the gay community for the startling effectiveness of its safer sex initiatives (King 1993). The fact that a senior police officer would make a public statement that was so at odds with the available evidence suggests that the lesbian and gay community may not get effective and equal protection from the police without a lot of continuing hard work on both sides.

Conclusion: some implications for professional practice

Social policy is a very complex area, and the provision of public services is inevitably fraught with conflict of all kinds. With a restricted pool of resources to meet growing need, questions of priority, rationing and the recognition of special needs are always likely to be contentious. Moreover, welfare provision is, by its very nature, always political. Because it involves the state spending public money, the policies and ideologies of political parties are inevitably bound up with decisions as to who gets what benefits and services, how much they get and who is responsible for administration and service provision (Ham 1992).

As public sector workers, health and social care professionals are inevitably affected by such issues, however much they may simply want to be allowed to get on with their jobs (George and Miller 1994; Ranade 1994). In terms of professional responsibility to lesbian or gay service users, there are two key implications of the policy issues discussed in this chapter. First, both an understanding of the degree to which sexuality is a factor in socio-political exclusion, and an acceptance that discrimination is still widely present in public service provision, become increasingly important in the context of interprofessional care management and delivery. Indeed, there are some circumstances in which the responsibility to provide effective care may well require the informed professional to take an active role in challenging such discrimination (Royal College of Nursing 1994; Wilton 1998).

There can be no doubt that social attitudes towards, and acceptance of, same-sex partnerships are improving (Annetts and Thompson 1992; Stonewall 1999). Stars such as George Michael, Rob Halford or Melissa

Etheridge have come out without damaging their careers, whilst countries as diverse as Canada, Australia, South Africa and Brazil have recognised the legitimacy of same-sex partnerships on at least some level. It can sometimes seem as if being gay is no longer a problem and well-meaning heterosexuals may not understand why some lesbians and gay men continue to agitate for political change. The second important lesson of this chapter, then, is that discrimination remains real, and that it has potentially serious consequences for anyone who happens to be lesbian or gay. In the interests of providing sensitive and appropriate care, health and social care professionals have a duty never to underestimate the social, psychological, emotional and even physiological effects that this long history of statutory discrimination may have on their clients.

exercises

Press and media

Over the next fortnight, note any press or media stories about homosexuality. You may wish to clip press articles and to video or take notes from television programmes or news items. Collect some stories from the gay press (*Gay Times, Diva, The Pink Paper*, etc.) for comparison. Now examine your collected items carefully:

- What is assumed about the audience or the reader?

- How many of the stories are written by a lesbian or gay man, or from a lesbian/gay-friendly perpective?

- What kind of language is used?

- What kind of images are presented?

- What overall image of lesbians and/or gay men is put across?

If you come across anything that is particularly offensive, you may wish to complain to the Press Complaints Commission at 1 Salisbury Square, London EC4Y 8AE, or the Broadcasting Standards Commission at 7 The Sanctuary, London SW1P 3JS.

Services

Collect together the Annual Reports of as many health and social care service providers as you can, in both the statutory and the voluntary sector. Housing associations, local charities, health care trusts, local authorities, youth groups, drugs projects and any organisation in receipt of public money should all produce annual reports and make them freely available.
  Examine them carefully.

- Do they mention lesbian, gay or bisexual service users?

- Do they offer any services to lesbians, gay men or bisexuals?

- What attempts do they make to liaise with the lesbian and gay community to assess their needs?

- Does their equal opportunities policy include reference to sexuality?

- Overall, what picture emerges of service provision to lesbians, gay men and bisexuals in your region?

- What are the likely consequences for your area of professional practice?

If you come across particularly glaring instances of omission, you may wish to write to the organisation concerned.

Further reading

Bock, G. and James, S. (eds) *Beyond Equality and Difference: Citizenship, Feminist Politics and Female Subjectivity*. London: Routledge.

Colvin, M. and Hawksley, J. (1989) *Section 28: A Practical Guide to the Law and its Implications*. London: Liberty.

Gonsiorek, J. and Weinrich, J. (eds) (1991) *Homosexuality: Research Implications for Public Policy*. London: Sage.

Kaufmann, T. and Lincoln, P. (eds) (1991) *High Risk Lives: Lesbian and Gay Politics after THE CLAUSE*. Bridport: The Prism Press.

Sanderson, T. (1995) *Mediawatch: The Treatment of Male and Female Homosexuality in the British Media*. London: Cassell.

Smith, A.M. (1994) *New Right Discourse on Race and Sexuality: Britain 1968–1990*. Cambridge: Cambridge University Press.

Tully, C. (1995) *Lesbian Social Services: Research Issues*. New York: Haworth Press.

10 sexuality and health promotion

Introduction

This chapter discusses health education and health promotion, both from a practical standpoint and from a more critical theoretical perspective drawing on the work of Michel Foucault. In practical terms, it assesses the difficulties inherent in promoting sexual health and identifies the assumptions that underly current health education practices in the targeting of sexual constituencies. This is followed by a discussion of health promotion as a discourse, and its contribution to social constructions of sexual orientation and sexual normality.

What is health promotion?

The terms 'health education' and 'health promotion' describe areas of activity that may overlap considerably, and are often confused with one another in public perception. However, it is important to understand some of their distinct characteristics if we are to disentangle the implications of sexuality for health promotion and vice versa.

Health education consists of activities designed to encourage people to cease activities thought to compromise their health, well-being or longevity and to adopt others believed to have health benefits. The aim of health education, according to *The Health of the Nation* (Department of Health 1992), is 'to ensure that individuals are able to exercise informed choice when selecting the lifestyle which they adopt'. But the notion that individuals are capable of 'selecting the lifestyles which they adopt' does not reflect the realities of most people's lives.

Although the consumerist rhetoric of glossy magazines may encourage the belief that anyone can 'select' the lifestyle of their choice, the ability to do so is restricted to a minority. Current public pronouncements on healthy living suggest that we should all eat plenty of organically grown fresh fruit and vegetables, base our diet around Mediterranean ingredients such as pasta, olive oil and a little red wine, exercise regularly, get plenty of sleep, and combat stress with plenty of relaxing holidays and a good balance of work and leisure. Such advice closely mirrors an affluent, white, middle-class 'lifestyle', but ignores the social and cultural factors that may restrict other people's ability to make such choices.

Given the opportunity, Black people would doubtless adopt a lifestyle free from the effects of racism; lesbians and gay men would abolish homophobia and pensioners would choose an adequate income. Unfortunately, such healthy choices are beyond individual control. It has long been recognised that simply giving people information about health does nothing to improve the cultural, structural, environmental, social and political factors that impact on the health of us all (Ewles and Simnett 1985; Aggleton 1990).

Health education also tends to reinforce the idea that biomedicine has the monopoly of 'correct' information about health and disease and that such information must be dispensed by authoritative experts. Whilst some health educators take great pains to encourage a more egalitarian practice, the very idea of professional health educators implies a 'top down' approach. As we shall see later, Foucault draws attention to this power relationship in his discussion of biopower. In the context of sexuality, this dependence on experts is likely to raise problems concerning the knowledge base and possible bias of the professionals concerned.

The individualistic focus of health education has also been criticised for its tendency towards victim-blaming. Anyone who does not follow expert advice is easily perceived as stubborn, ignorant or incompetent, with illness the inevitable consequence of personal weakness (Lupton 1995). It was awareness of problems of this kind that led, in part, to the development of *health promotion* in the 1970s. The term itself was first used by the then

Canadian Minister of National Health and Welfare, Marc Lalonde, who argued that social and psychological factors played an important part in preventing illness and enhancing health. This approach has been reflected in the shift in emphasis from curative medicine to preventative primary health care, which underpins the World Health Organization (WHO) strategy aiming for 'Health For All by the Year 2000'.

The goal of health promotion has been summarised as 'to make the healthy choice the easy choice' (Naidoo and Wills 1994). To this end it is recognised that every level of society must be involved, from national governments to local employers and from international agencies to families. As expressed by WHO, the aim is 'to ensure that the total environment, which is beyond the control of individuals, is conducive to health'. Four fundamental prerequisites for such an environment have been identified (WHO 1985, cited in Naidoo and Wills 1994: 75):

1 Peace and freedom from the fear of war.
2 Equal opportunity for all and social justice.
3 Satisfaction of basic needs.
4 Political commitment and public support.

Health *promotion* is therefore a broader and more ambitious enterprise than health *education* alone. Health promotion interventions may include everything from legislation to the development of new technologies, from employment policies to workplace practices. Although health education is likely to be ineffective on its own in promoting sustainable behaviour change, it does remain one of the key tools of health promotion. As we shall see, sexual orientation is a significant issue in both health education and health promotion.

Barriers to health: homophobia

Since the WHO has identified equal opportunity and social justice as key components of health promotion, this suggests that homophobia and heterosexism are incompatible with the goal of developing a healthy, health-promoting society. Indeed, there is a strong argument for regarding homophobia as symptomatic of social 'dis-ease', since it has been found to be associated with high levels of anxiety and insecurity in homophobic individuals themselves, as well as in those likely to experience discrimination as a result (Kitzinger 1987; Greenberg 1988; Mason and Palmer 1997).

If we accept the holistic model of health proposed by WHO, it seems unlikely that homophobia would flourish in a society which provided effective support to ensure the sexual health and well-being of all its members. Indeed, there is much evidence to suggest that countries which have the most relaxed and tolerant attitudes towards their lesbian and gay citizens – such as the Netherlands, Denmark and Sweden – are also characterised by lower levels of sexual violence, teenage pregnancies and other indicators of sexual dis-ease (International Lesbian and Gay Association 1988; Tatchell 1990; Griffin and Mulholland 1997; Macionis and Plummer 1997). High levels of homophobia appear to be symptomatic of a social environment that is unhealthy for all its citizens, gay or straight. This suggests the need to explore more theoretical approaches to health promotion. One such approach, which is particularly relevant in the context of sexuality, is that of the influential French theorist Michel Foucault.

A radical critique: Foucault's concept of biopower

Foucault, himself openly gay, developed a rigorous analysis of medicine as an apparatus of social control, a critique that has implications for the promotion of health. Two elements in particular are especially relevant to an understanding of human sexuality in the context of health promotion. First, he developed the idea of a particular form of power, *disciplinary power*, and demonstrated the means through which it operates in industrialised societies. In his analysis, medicine is probably the single most important axis of this disciplinary power. Second, he was the first thinker of such stature to foreground the question of sexuality in his discussions of political power, and to identify the ways in which sexuality is exploited in the interests of social control.

Earlier thinkers, such as Sigmund Freud or Wilhelm Reich, assumed that social control was achieved and maintained by simply repressing sexuality, and presented the familiar picture of civilised societies struggling to contain the unruly impulses of desire and eroticism. Foucault challenged this, insisting that disciplinary power goes hand in hand with an 'incitement' to sexuality and with the widespread expectation that we will all 'confess' our sexual secrets regularly in a variety of contexts, from the Catholic confessional to the doctor's surgery to the television chat show (Foucault 1976). His analysis was not complete; he has been widely criticised, for example, for failing to take the power relations of gender into account, However, others have been able to apply his conceptual framework to an examination of gender and of other issues that he himself neglected.

Foucault coined the terms 'biopower', 'biopolitics' and 'anatamo-politics' to describe the ways in which he believed disciplinary power operated in society. We all have bodies, and the exercise of social power must inevitably include power over bodies. Hence, 'biopower' refers to the structural mechanisms whereby whole populations are managed and individuals are disciplined. These include not only familiar control mechanisms, such as prisons and police cells (which restrain the bodies of criminals and suspected criminals), but also hospitals, schools, residential care units, old people's homes, etc. The concept has been useful in identifying the ways in which women and men are disciplined in different ways by gender roles; it is possible, for example, to regard the fashion industry as exercising biopower in its insistence that women must be very thin in order to be socially acceptable (Eckermann 1997). The approach has also been used to criticise the pharmaceutical industry's promotion of hormone replacement therapy (HRT) for all menopausal women (Gullette 1997; Harding 1997).

There are two aspects to biopower, the 'biopolitics of the population', which is organised around regulatory controls and measurements (such as demographic statistics) and 'the anatamo-politics of the human body', which refers to the 'integration [of the body] into systems of efficient and economic controls' (Foucault 1976: 139). The debate surrounding the use of these terms is complex, and cannot be presented in detail here. However, it is clear that Foucault and his followers have developed a critical perspective which has much to offer in the analysis of health and health promotion practice.

From a Foucauldian perspective, 'health education can make a contribution to the exercise of bio-power because it deals with norms of healthy behaviours and promotes discipline for the achievement of good health' (Gastaldo 1997: 113). It encourages individuals to discipline themselves, urging them to use their bodies in ways that the experts have deemed to be acceptable and 'good'.

In the long run, then, one effect of health education and health care is to reinforce the power of biomedicine. Both work by enabling biomedicine to gain certain forms of access to people's bodies and lives. It is seen as acceptable for individuals to be interviewed, weighed, measured, tested and observed in the interests of protecting the health of themselves and of the wider population. Indeed, notions of discipline are widespread in both health education and health and social care practice. We expect patients to submit with docility to the treatments prescribed by doctors, however painful or unpleasant they may be. Social workers often encourage particular forms of discipline (alcohol avoidance, restraint from antisocial behaviour, etc.) in their clients in order to achieve specified case outcomes. So:

> The political space that health care and policy constitute is an important site for the exercise of disciplinary power. Focusing on individual bodies or on the social body, health professionals are entitled by scientific knowledge/power to examine, interview and prescribe 'healthy' lifestyles.
>
> (Gastaldo 1997: 116)

None of the above implies that health and social care interventions are not good and desirable. A patient whose illness is cured as a result of disciplined submission to medical power benefits enormously. Nevertheless, it remains important to recognise that power is one of the key issues in the practice of health and social care, and of health education in particular. 'Health education,' writes Gastaldo (1997: 118), 'is an experience of being governed from the outside and a request for self-discipline . . . [it] is a constructive exercise of power . . . through the promotion of health it circulates everywhere in spheres that are new to biomedicine.'

Biopower and sexuality

In our exploration of the relationship between sexuality and health promotion, Foucault's concept of biopower offers an additional perspective, enabling us to ask new questions of health educators and policy makers. Foucault identified both sexuality and medical power as central elements of disciplinary power in contemporary industrialised societies. This should alert us to the possibility of the control of sexualities through health and social care, and should influence our interpretation of official discourse on such topics as single parents, the age of consent and lesbian and gay families. Clearly, the practice of health educators is likely to be especially significant here.

Promoting sexual health in practice

The practice of promoting sexual health tends, in general, to mean the prevention of sexually transmissible diseases, but just as health means more than the absence of disease or infirmity so too sexual health means more than freedom from STDs. WHO identifies three elements of sexual health (cited in Naidoo and Wills 1994: 239):

1 The capacity to enjoy and express sexuality without guilt or shame in fulfilling emotional relationships.
2 The capacity to control fertility.
3 Freedom from disorders which compromise health and sexual or reproductive function.

Those whose professional practice brings them into daily contact with the sick, injured, distressed or socially excluded are probably better placed than most to recognise the extent to which sexual health is bound up with general health and well-being.

The nursing model

From a nursing perspective, Webb (1985) identifies nine key aspects of a nurse's responsibility for sexual health promotion with patients. Nurses should be able to:

1 initiate discussion with patients regarding their sexual health (for example, following major surgery)
2 respond to patients' requests for information about sexual health concerns (for example, safer sex techniques)
3 reassure patients that their sexual health concerns are normal and natural
4 teach patients about the effects of disease or trauma on their sexual health (for example, following brain injury, strokes or certain cancers)

5 teach patients about the possible effects of therapeutic interventions on their sexual health (for example, following gynaecological surgery or when a colostomy is required)

6 counsel patients who experience a change in their self-concept relating to sexual health (for example, following mastectomy, clinically induced menopause or removal of the prostate)

7 teach patients adaptive approaches to sexual expression (for example, after damage to the central nervous system or in progressively debilitating disease)

8 fulfil the role of patient advocate in relation to sexual health concerns (for example, by gathering information, locating support groups, etc.)

9 refer patients who are experiencing sexual health problems to appropriate personnel (for example, by arranging appointments with GUM clinics or specialist lesbian or gay sexual health clinics).

This is an enormously taxing list! It is hardly surprising that nurses in Britain feel ill-equipped to fulfill this aspect of their role. One recent survey found that nurse training fails to provide nurses with the knowledge base and interpersonal skills which must underpin sexual health promotion and that nurses' ability to discuss sexual health with patients was extremely inhibited. Factors identified by nurses in this study included embarrassment, concern about the reaction of patients or colleagues, lack of knowledge and 'discomfort in discussions with patients, particularly with patients of the opposite sex to the nurse, or of homosexual orientation' (Barrett 1997: 52).

Female nurses have long struggled against the stereotypical (hetero)-sexualisation of their role, and some continue to wage daily battle against sexual harassment from colleagues and male patients. Male nurses, on the other hand, have to contend with the assumption that any man entering such a feminised occupation must be gay. Of course, a proportion are, but, as Savage comments (1987: 76), 'a proportion of female nurses are lesbians without this becoming the predominant stereotype'. Sexuality and gender issues are therefore likely to be experienced by nurses as problematic issues in terms of professional identity. The extremely intimate nature of the contact between nurses and patients introduces a further element of anxiety associated with the need to ensure that nurse–patient interactions are firmly held within the bounds of a professional relationship whose nature is understood by both parties. It is therefore not surprising that Barrett's research found that nurses avoided broaching the subject of sexual health with patients out of 'Concern that patients would react with embarrassment, interpret a discussion on sexual health as an intrusion on privacy, or respond to the nurse as a sexual being rather than as a professional practitioner' (Barret 1997: 56).

Social care issues

Although the professional contact between nurses and their patients involves unique elements of physical intimacy, similar issues confront other health care professionals and arise in social work, community work and some aspects of youth work. Undue intimacy between worker and client is a persistent concern, which 'comes with the territory'. The potential for inappropriate sexual contact is something that health and social care professionals are (rightly) encouraged to be vigilant against, and the professional consequences of crossing the boundary of what is acceptable – or even of being *perceived* to have done so – can be disastrous. The requirement to initiate discussion of sex and sexuality in the interests of promoting sexual health can therefore lead to anxiety about compromising professional boundaries.

The question of minority sexualities can cause additional stress. Research indicates that the majority of those working in health and social care are ill-informed about issues affecting the well-being of their lesbian and gay clients and/or are actively hostile towards this group (Stevens 1993; Annesley 1995; Hardman 1996; Wilton 1997b). Training and education about professionally relevant lesbian and gay issues is extremely sparse, even for doctors; one typical survey of medical curricula in the US found that the average time devoted to the topic of homosexuality was slightly over three hours *in total* over a four-year training course (Singer and Deschamps 1994: 39).

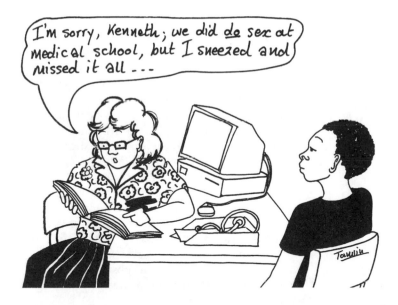

It seems that, with the exception of some specialist units, very little sexual health promotion of any kind is carried out in health and social care settings. If and when it does, many practitioners are ill-prepared by their training, de-skilled by general lack of clarity about their role as sexual health advocates, and likely to experience feelings of vulnerability, anxiety and embarrassment. Homophobic attitudes and widespread failure to address lesbian and gay sexual health issues in training mean that the needs of this group are particularly unlikely to be met.

Target audiences

Outwith the professional environments where interactions between professional and client are formalised – hospitals, secure units, residential care centres, etc. – health educators also attempt to promote the health of the public at large. To do this they employ a range of strategies, including leafleting campaigns, press adverts, mobile information units or mass media campaigns. In addition, certain 'captive audiences' in places such as schools, antenatal clinics, youth clubs, universities and health care waiting areas may be targeted with sexual health information. However, professional health educators are not the sole source of health information. Indeed, they probably produce *less* health information and advice than the commercial sector, in the form of 'Health and Beauty' sections in popular magazines, or advertisements for health care products.

Whether produced by health professionals or commercial advertisers, such campaigns are carefully targeted. This is the case for health information generally, but it is especially evident where sexual health is concerned. There is a recognition that different social groups may have very different requirements in terms of information and advice, and that cultural attitudes to sexuality and sexual practices vary widely.

Health-related behaviours and sexuality

The key concerns of health educators (alcohol and substance use, diet, sexual health and exercise) are all areas in which people's behaviour is likely to be influenced by their sexuality. For example, heterosexual women's attitude to exercise has been shown to be strongly associated with anxieties about their attractiveness to men (Cameron *et al.* 1996), which is probably not the case for lesbians. Although lesbians are not, of course, insulated from prevailing notions of female attractiveness, there are specific ideals of attractiveness within lesbian subcultures (Burana *et al.* 1994; Jay 1995; Halberstam and Volcano 1999). This is likely to affect the kinds of exercise that both groups of women choose and this, in turn, may lead to different implications for physical and emotional well-being. Similarly, gay men are likely to be much better informed than their heterosexual peers about safer sexual practices, but are also more likely to experience problems with substance over-use (Shernoff and Scott 1988), making it important to tailor health information accordingly.

Families

The notion of the family is key to the social organisation of sexuality and is particularly significant to public health. Health educators tend to work with a particular set of assumptions about the role of women as wives and mothers. As a result, it is they who are given information about healthy eating, safety in the home and other such issues, because they are expected to take responsibility for safeguarding the health of their partners and children. As Deborah Lupton (1996: 119) concludes:

> contemporary health promotion campaigns tend to place the emphasis of responsibility for health promotion upon women, in their role as wives and mothers . . . Women are expected to regulate the diet of their partners and offspring according to the dictates of health guidelines, to monitor their partner's weight and exercise habits, to ensure the cleanliness of their children . . . and to desist from smoking and alcohol consumption during pregnancy and even afterwards.

Lupton and others criticise this approach for allowing men to absolve themselves of responsibility and for presenting women's health as of secondary importance to that of their families (Doyal 1995; Lupton 1996; Wilton 1997a). What is less often acknowledged is that lesbian and gay families, step-families, single-parent families and others are not well served by a model of family health that remains closely tied to narrow concepts of domestic gender relations.

Heterosexuality, although entirely taken for granted in this context, remains unacknowledged. This can lead to a situation whereby health education reinforces a particular relationship that women have with the state. As Lupton found (1996: 119), 'since the nineteenth century public health strategies have traditionally represented women as mothers, the guardians of their families' health, and by extension, that of the nation's, and have targeted them for intervention as agents of regulation'.

Since lesbians and gay men are excluded from the accepted notion of what constitutes a family, it is not surprising that this affects the way they are addressed by health educators. Lesbians and gay men are usually targeted as people living *outside* family structures, with a focus on health issues typically associated with the lifestyle of the urban gay 'scene', such as alcohol or substance abuse and AIDS awareness.

Such initiatives are clearly to be welcomed. However, lesbian and gay lifestyles are as varied as those of heterosexuals. There is, therefore, a difficult balance to strike between responding to the health consequences of lifestyles that revolve around the 'scene', and focusing on those to the exclusion of others whose needs may be less visible. By addressing lesbians and gay target groups *as if* they all conformed to a particular stereotype, health educational discourse itself contributes to the credibility of the stereotype. These and other unintended consequences of health education practice are discussed in the next section.

Discourses of health

Besides its use in everyday speech, 'discourse' is also a technical term used by poststructuralists and other critical theorists (Weedon 1987; Fraser 1989). Since it is often misunderstood, a brief outline will be given here. Nick Fox defines 'discourse' as; 'Written, spoken or enacted practices organized so as to supply a coherent claim to a position or perspective' (Fox

1993: 161). Clearly not all 'written, spoken or enacted practices' count; they must be recognised as meaningful, and are often accompanied by claims to some form of authority. Jennifer Harding's definition of medical discourse is also useful: 'By "medical discourse" I mean what is said by those speaking as medical experts, and which locates them as such, in a clinical setting, a lecture hall or on the printed page' (Harding 1997: 148).

However, questions of authority and expertise are not necessarily clear cut. As we have seen, health educational discourse is produced in a variety of locations; some of it comes from professionally trained health educators, doctors, medical researchers or other recognised 'experts', but some is produced by journalists, advertising copywriters, self-help organisations and others. Clearly the authority that these different parties can claim has very different foundations, and they may each bring quite different kinds of expertise to their role. Health educational discourse therefore reflects many different kinds of knowledge, and may well be internally conflictual or contradictory.

Discourse and reality

The reason for examining health educational discourse is that it enables us to understand some of its unintended consequences. Discourses do not simply reflect pre-existing reality, they actively contribute to the construction of reality as we experience it (Sarup 1993; Chaplin 1994). To use the jargon, 'social constructs are discursively produced'. And, as we have learned already, social constructs (such as 'body' or 'femininity') are the product of so many social interactions that they tend to be fluid and changing.

Some of the discursive elements that go to make up a social construct such as femininity are produced with quite deliberate intent. The fashion and cosmetics industries, for example, are aware that it is in their interests to be accepted as an authoritative voice defining femininity, and to be able to change that definition in order to get women to spend money on their products. However, other practices (such as health education) have very different aims. Here, the contribution to the social construction of femininity may be an unintended – indeed, even unknowing – consequence of their activities.

When, for example, health educators launch an anti-smoking campaign targeting young women, they may not be aware that their campaign will inevitably contribute to the social construction of what a young woman is. However, such messages may be powerful precisely because they come from an authoritative source which is perceived as disinterested.

As inhabitants of a very media-aware society, most individuals are probably sophisticated enough to recognise that commercial interests are out to manipulate us in order to get their hands on our money. Health educators, in contrast, are assumed to be acting altruistically. This means that audiences are more likely to interpret health educational materials as reflecting the 'real world'. Moreover, since medical discourse is one of the most powerful and influential – indeed, many argue that it is *the* most powerful (Petersen and Bunton 1997) – any discourse that is associated with medicine tends to bathe in the reflected glow of that power (Fox 1993; Gullette 1997).

Constructing sexual normality

Discourses contribute to social construction in many ways. These include *representation*, the ways in which a topic is written or spoken about and the visual imagery associated with it; *silence* or *absence*, the lack of attention paid to certain topics, which indicates that they are unimportant or shameful, or even that they do not exist; *proliferation*, the excessive attention paid to topics, which gives the impression that they are extremely important; and *address*, by which is meant the sometimes unspoken assumptions about who comprises the intended readership or audience for a particular text (for more detail on these elements, see Weedon 1987; Fraser 1989; Chaplin 1994; Wilton 1997a). These elements are each important on their own but, by examining how they act together, we can develop a critical understanding of the ways in which a discourse contributes to the construction of social reality.

Both medical texts and popular books on sex have, until very recently, written of homosexuality as a problem or deviation from the norm (see, for example, Jennings White 1925; Reuben 1969; Comfort 1972; Calderone and Johnson 1989). In so doing they are *representing* homosexuality as a disordered sexuality. The medical profession is regarded as having specialist knowledge about sexual function, and many books on sex aimed at a general readership are at pains to stress their medical credentials, so this representation is very influential.

On the other hand, midwifery texts routinely ignore the requirements of lesbians when discussing antenatal care, with the consequence that the idea 'lesbian' becomes *absent* from the social construct 'expectant mother' (see, for example, Symonds and Hunt 1996). This gives tacit encouragement to the idea that lesbians cannot or should not be mothers, and because midwifery is an authoritative discourse on mothering, this carries considerable weight as a contribution to the social construction of both 'mother' and 'lesbian'.

Discursive absence also works in a quite different way, with some groups tending to be absent from discourses of sexuality altogether. Elderly or disabled lesbians and gay men, for example, have long complained that they are a particularly invisible and ill-served minority in literature on sexuality or sexual health (Shernoff and Scott 1988; Deevey 1990; Lynch and Woods 1996; Shakespeare *et al.* 1996).

On the other hand, gay men are mentioned with disproportionate frequency in specialist texts dealing with HIV/AIDS (see, for example, Institute of Medicine 1986; Kirkpatrick and Kirkpatrick 1987; Shilts 1987). This is, of course, a complex issue, since there is a real need to recognise the specific problems of gay men. However, in the context of HIV, this *proliferation* of references to gay men and disease adds great weight to the belief that gay sex is intrinsically unhealthy.

The problems of *address* are often subtle. In 1986, for example, the British government issued a leaflet to every household in the country giving advice about preventing HIV transmission. The front cover proclaimed that 'More people are dying of AIDS every month and they are *not* only gay men and drug users. This leaflet tells you how to protect yourself.' This wording implied that the leaflet was *addressed* to people who were *not* 'homosexuals or drug addicts'. This reinforced the impression that these groups were not included in the 'general public' and that they were completely cut off from the normal, everyday sort of person who was likely to live in a household and read the leaflet. Moreover, as Watney points out (1987), the use of the word 'only' can be read as implying that infections among gay men and drug users are unimportant.

Whilst each example may be innocuous on its own, taken together they contribute very powerfully to the social construct of lesbians and gay men as social outcasts who are associated with disease and do not do the sorts of things that 'normal' people do, like have babies or take steps to protect themselves from becoming sick. Since these texts base their claims to authority on some form of close relationship with medicine, they are seen as constituent parts of medical discourse. Thus, detailed critique of their representations, absences and proliferations, as well as their assumptions about address, demonstrates the role of medical discourse in the social construction of homosexuality as abnormal and marginal (Patton 1985; Watney 1987; Kayal 1993; Terry and Urla 1995; Waldby 1996; Rosario 1997; Wilton 1997a).

Deconstructing homosexuality: an example

Discourse analysis is an immensely complex task. However, it is useful if it enables the producers of discourse to assess the unintended consequences of their actions, and to take responsibility for them. Even when health educators are working from the best possible motives, and are drawing on the community knowledge of local lesbians and gay men there are many pitfalls. This can be demonstrated by a detailed deconstruction of two leaflets produced by the Alcohol Advisory Service and Lesbian and Gay Switchboard in Hereford and Worcester (Figure 10.1).

The leaflet addressed to gay men has the headline, 'What's long, hard and round and can be a source of both pleasure and pain?' The front cover then opens to reveal . . . a bottle of lager. Of course the reader's mind is supposed to supply the answer 'a penis', in the long-established tradition of comic innuendo. The lesbian leaflet, on the other hand, asks 'Is your best friend called Stella?' When this leaflet is opened, it continues 'or Margherita? Or Sherry? Or Bloody Mary?'

Puns on women's names are less of a 'dirty' joke than the penis–bottle innuendo. However, think a little about the implications of these very

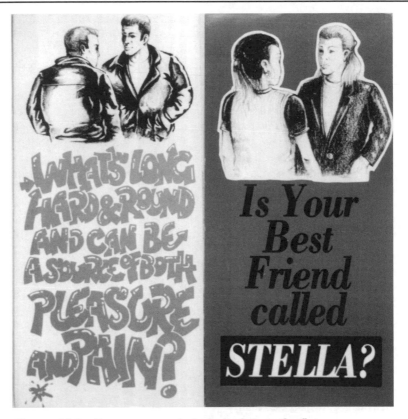

Figure 10.1 Front covers of alcohol advisory leaflets.

different forms of address. Gay men are being addressed with a joke which is unavoidably sexual, to the point of being a little shocking. There is nothing here about relationships, names or people, just a penis. Lesbians are not being asked about sex or lovers, they are being asked about their *best friend*; the stress is on relationships and names, with nothing at all about anything sexual.

For textual deconstruction to be meaningful, material cannot be examined in isolation. Taken out of context, little can be said about these leaflets. However, if they are examined in the broader context of the social construction of lesbian and gay male sexuality, something emerges which is troubling. Gay men have traditionally been constructed as primarily sexual, uninterested in intimacy or relationships, concerned only with penises and not with the people attached to them (Dyer 1989; Edwards 1994; Wilton 1997a), a stereotype not borne out by research into actual behaviours (Singer and Deschamps 1994). In contrast, lesbians have been constructed as childlike, uninterested in sex, seeking emotional intimacy, or mothering over adult sexuality, and their relationships with their lovers have been dismissed as nothing more than very close friendships (Scruton 1986; Smith 1992; Wilton 1997a). These jokey leaflets have the unintended consequence of reinforcing such stereotypes.

Let us follow this train of thought one stage further and ask, do notions such as these *promote health* for lesbians or for gay men? Is it in the interests of gay men that those providing services to them, or indeed they themselves, should believe that gay men are only interested in sex? What are the likely consequences for a young man, just coming to terms with being gay and looking desperately for a supportive peer group, if he is led to believe that being gay is all about 'what's long, hard and round'? Is it is the interests of lesbians if their most important relationships are dismissed as immature and not to be taken as seriously as adult heterosexual relationships?

It may seem that this is an awful lot of fuss to make about two leaflets. Indeed, it is; and in the absence of other efforts to educate lesbians and gay men about safer drinking habits, the fact that this campaign exists at all must be applauded. However, it is only by a detailed analysis of this kind that health educators are able to spot the particular contribution that their work makes to the social construction of sexualities. It is not only sexuality that is at issue here. Unintended messages about gender, race, age, disability and other social variables also require careful assessment (Gilman 1995; McClintock 1995; Terry and Urla 1995). However, because sexuality still goes unrecognised as a significant issue in health promotion, it is particularly important to draw attention to it.

Deconstructing heterosexuality

By constructing lesbian and gay sexualities so narrowly, health educational discourse has a tangential impact on the construction of heterosexuality. Summarising her research into 'discourses about human sexuality in the medical and public health literature', Deborah Lupton concludes:

> gay men . . . are typically represented as enjoying multiple casual sexual encounters, always involving anal penetration; heterosexual men are positioned as experiencing uncontrollable sexual urges, constantly frustrated by their female partners in their attempts to have sex as often as possible . . . Hence, those men who may not necessarily be very often interested in sex, come to view themselves as aberrant, needing therapy or medical treatment.
>
> (Lupton 1996: 88–9)

Inevitably, discourses that position 'men' in a particular way with regard to sex also establish a position for 'women' by implication. Thus, the female partner constantly frustrating men's desire for frequent sex constitutes a specific norm for heterosexual female behaviour, one which consists of avoiding sexual contact and taking control of and responsibility for heterosexual relations. These polarised positions for male and female sexuality within discourses of heterosex have troubling implications for the ability of women and men to negotiate sexual encounters and relationships in ways that promote their emotional and physical well-being (Berer with Ray 1993; Wilton 1997a; Foreman 1999).

Within the context of heterosexuality, the construction of women's sexuality in medical discourse is especially troubling (see Treichler 1988). Think critically, for example, about the implications of this statement, which was written by a leading expert in reproductive biology and included as part of the editorial to the Medical Research Council's quarterly magazine:

> What new preventive strategies do we need to put in place to protect and preserve reproductive health? Whatever we do must be implemented in adolescence . . . The monumental study by Anne Johnson and her colleagues of sexual behaviour in Britain showed that . . . whereas boys tended to be the same age as their first sexual partners, 75 per cent of the girls had had first sex with older men. *This makes the girls the group most likely to introduce sexually transmitted diseases into their adolescent cohort.*
>
> (Short 1997: 1, my emphasis)

What is happening in this passage? First, note how 'the girls' have become separated out from 'their cohort'. They are the ones seen as 'most likely to introduce STDs' *into* that cohort; they become wandering beings who have 'left' and then return bearing an unwanted extra from *outside*. With the girls separated out in this way, 'the cohort' that remains consists entirely of boys. Second, note how the 'older men' who are in fact *responsible* for infecting 'the girls' with STDs are rendered absent or invisible as responsible agents. It would be more reasonable to state that 'older men who have sex with young women are responsible for introducing STDs into the adolescent cohort', but this is not how the situation is presented to us.

Finally, note that the health of 'the girls' is *at no time* foregrounded as a concern in its own right. Professor Short fails to draw our attention to the consequences for these girls of being infected with an STD by an older man; rather he deflects attention away from them on to the 'cohort' (that is, boys of their own age) to whom they may 'introduce' STDs. By absolving the older men in this way and by presenting 'the girls' as dangerous to their 'cohort' rather than at risk themselves, two meanings are implied: (1) that our primary concern must be with the health of the boys, and (2) that it is the girls who are the culpable group in this unhappy scenario. The 'cohort' is presented as free from STDs until they are 'introduced' by the girls.

Nor is there any acknowledgement of the differentials in power that may exist between the girls and these older men. We are told simply that 'the girls . . . had sex' with them. In the wider context of what we know about gender and heterosex, this is a rather strange reversal of general practice. It is far more usual to speak of men 'having sex with' women, since it is by and large men who have the freedom to choose their sexual partners, to take the initiative in sexual encounters, and to dictate what kinds of activity take place. Heterosex is most frequently presented as something that men 'do to' women (Segal 1994; Richardson 1996; Wilton 1997a). We know that the degree of power that young women exercise over their early sexual relationships is relatively limited (Gavey 1992; Stewart 1996). It is therefore less than responsible to present their sexual encounters with older men without acknowledging such imbalances of power and identifying coercion as a potential factor.

Once more, it has required a lengthy and detailed critical analysis of an apparently simple statement to dig out the troubling implications. Why bother? Given the disproportionate influence that medical discourse has in the social construction of genders and sexualities, there is a corresponding duty for practitioners to be reflexive, to identify unintended consequences such as these and to take responsibility for correcting their practice accordingly. The conclusion of the piece we are discussing is that:

> What is needed is some concerted action by the various government departments and other bodies involved in health education to ensure that safe sex education becomes a mandatory part of every school curriculum, so that the theory is taught *before* the practice begins . . . Safe sex education in school is the best investment that any country could make to ensure the long-term reproductive health of its people.
>
> (Short 1997: 1)

This is a laudable aim, and one which AIDS activists and many other groups have been trying to achieve in this country for many years (Aggleton and Homans 1987; King *et al.* 1989; Aggleton *et al.* 1990; National AIDS Trust 1991; World Health Organization 1992). However, it is only part of the conclusion that must be drawn from the evidence presented by Professor Short. School-based education in safe sex is not going to be particularly effective with those 'older men'. Nor is it going to be of much use to 'the girls', since study after study has shown that, however well-informed they may be, they have very little power to insist that their male partners practise safer sex (Richardson 1989; Panos Institute 1990; Gavey 1992; Berer with Ray 1993; Stewart 1996).

The article is intended to contribute to the *protection* of young people from STDs. However, because it (albeit unwittingly) contributes to the construction of young women's sexual activity as dangerous to men (rather than the other way round), its author has been unable to identify that the most significant risk factor in terms of adolescent sexual health is *not* the sexual behaviour of 'the girls' but that of adult men. Devising sexual health promotional strategies in response to this requires much more than safe sex education for adolescents. Discourse analysis is an extremely useful technique to employ when developing more effective approaches.

Conclusion

Health education discourse relies on the construction of agreed definitions of 'health' and 'normality'. However, it is clear that any such constructs are likely to contribute to processes of social inclusion and exclusion. Those who are perceived as 'choosing' unhealthy or 'abnormal' behaviours or lifestyles risk being blamed for their illnesses or being socially marginalised (much as some smokers' groups claim has been done to them). Moreover, if certain attributes are represented in health educational discourse as 'normal' or 'healthy', whatever is presented as the 'opposite' to that becomes the negatively valued 'other', which must be rejected by those who wish to be seen as normal and healthy.

It may be one unintended consequence of health educational discourse, as we have seen, to construct very specific and narrowly defined sexualities as healthy whilst constructing others as abnormal or unhealthy. Those 'other' sexualities then become something to be rejected and disparaged by anyone who seeks normality and health.

However, it is important not to become too conspiratorial here. The subtle forms of power identified by a Foucauldian analysis are so pervasive that most of us seldom recognise them, any more than a fish recognises the water in which it swims. They are a condition of life in complex societies, and most politicians take them as much for granted as the rest of us. However, the notion of reflexive practice, and the demands of a model of care based on human need, mean that those who are responsible for exercising these forms of power – and that includes everyone working in the health and social care professions – take as much responsibility as they are able for exercising it ethically and with awareness.

Every health educational intervention has potential consequences for the social construction of sexualities and of genders. So too does every health or social care environment. Lupton concludes that this is particularly troubling, since it means that these important public services may be unable to meet the diverse needs of the populations which they are supposed to serve:

> the insistence on discriminating between men/women, active/passive, the masculine/the feminine, Self/Other and disciplined/unruly has been central to medical and public health discourses and remains so. Such essentialisms are too reductive, failing to recognize the plurality of difference that exists in the social world.
>
> (Lupton 1996: 159)

As we have seen, such practices are problematic not only because they fail to take account of diversity, but also because they contribute to the social exclusion of groups defined in these discourses as 'Other'.

exercise

Over the next week collect together as many examples of health education as possible. You may find leaflets in clinic waiting areas, GPs' surgeries, supermarkets and pharmacies, as well as articles and adverts in magazines or practice journals (such as *Nursing Times* or *Social Work Today*). The free papers posted to GPs every week contain large numbers of adverts from drugs companies, which are a useful source if you have access to them. You could also usefully video all the adverts or programmes relating to health that you come across in a week's television viewing.

Either alone or working in a small group, analyse the material you have gathered using the following criteria:

Representation: How does each piece represent people of different sexualities? Does it contain photographs, images, illustrations or cartoons, which imply heterosexual or homosexual relationships? What emotional states are associated with images of people – joy, fun, sadness, etc., and how do these states relate to sexuality? What about families? Are there any images or words that make it possible for the audience to imagine that families could be anything other than heterosexual?

Silence/absence: Which groups are absent from these materials? What kinds of people are *not* written about or depicted in pictures, images, etc.? Think about age, ethnicity and disability in the context of sexuality as well as heterosexuals and gay people.

Proliferation: Which groups are presented most often, and in what context? What images are used most frequently, and what is the effect of this? What kinds of 'norm', if any, are being suggested by these materials?

Address: What assumptions are being made about the audience? Are any of the materials overtly 'targeted', and if so, at which groups and why? Are there any unintended consequences of this targeting? Are there assumptions about the gender of the audience, and what are these assumptions?

When you have carried out this thorough analysis, try to draw some conclusions in answer to this research question: 'How do these materials contribute to the social construction of genders and sexualities?' Then move on to the final stage of the research, 'What might the consequences be for the health of different groups?'

Note: While you are doing this exercise you may find yourself working hard to 'force' certain images to work in a certain way. For example, you may want to suggest that a picture of a woman with a baby on her own 'could' be interpreted as a picture of a lesbian with a baby. If you find yourself doing this, ask yourself two questions, 'Why am I doing this?' and 'Given what I know about the culture that produced these materials, how realistic am I being?' The answers to these questions are just as important in terms of your personal awareness as the exercise itself.

Further reading

Lupton, D. (1996) *The Imperative of Health: Public Health and the Regulated Body*. London: Sage.

Petersen, A. and Bunton, R. (eds) (1997) *Foucault, Health and Medicine*. London: Routledge.

Shakespeare, T., Gillespie-Sells, K. and Davies, D. (eds) (1996) *The Sexual Politics of Disability: Untold Desires*. London: Cassell.

Turner, B.S. (1995) *Medical Power and Social Knowledge*. London: Sage.

Wilton, T. (1997) *En/Gendering AIDS: Deconstructing Sex, Text and Epidemic*. London: Sage.

11 moving towards good practice

Introduction

Health and social care is, by its very nature, a rapidly changing field, as new developments in therapies, treatments and forms of support are fed through into practice. Practitioners are also required to respond rapidly to policy directives. Since frequent change is such an occupational hazard, it is perhaps not surprising that there may be a degree of inertia, or even resistance, to changes in the wider society, unless they are clearly relevant to practice. This may in part account for findings that, in basic training, knowledge, attitudes and practices to do with sexuality lag behind what is required for good practice.

The speed of response to particular issues also varies between the professions. Social work, for example, has led the field in anti-discriminatory practice, but has been slower in extending this to include sexuality. Nursing, on the other hand, which has not traditionally been perceived as a trailblazing profession, has taken some very important initiatives in setting anti-homophobic standards of care, although there is little evidence that the issue is adequately covered in training (Cossis Brown 1992; Royal College of Nursing 1994).

In a climate of increasing intersectorial collaboration, the importance of multidisciplinary care teams is growing. The current interest in 'holism', and critical recognition of the limits of a segregated approach to health and well-being means that the days of professional territorialism in the organisation and delivery of care are numbered (Gabe *et al.* 1994; George and Miller 1994). The interface between health care and social care is becoming ever more permeable, so that it becomes ever more important to establish basic standards of care across the entire professional field.

This chapter aims to contribute to the development of such standards by discussing current practice issues to do with sexuality, summarising current research findings and locating them in their historical and socio-cultural context, examining some of the problems facing researchers in the field, and outlining some key examples of good practice. Attention is also given to the practicalities of improving practice, on both an individual and institutional level. Clearly, topics such as these could easily fill a book by themselves, so the chapter concludes with a substantial resources section to support ongoing developmental work.

Moving forward: new developments

Practice developments cannot, of course, take place in a vacuum. Rather, they need to be underpinned by a sound framework of theory and empirical research. Nor is it necessarily a simple matter to put research into practice. To do this requires effective channels for the dissemination of relevant research findings within the various professions engaged in health and social care. Existing beliefs and attitudes may need to be challenged and, in the case of sexuality, this may be a time-consuming process. In a straitened economic climate, with fierce competition for research funding and practice budgets, the question of resources may also be a stumbling block.

What follows is a discussion of current key issues in theory, research and practice developments which can contribute to better practice in this area, starting with an overview of the issues that confront researchers.

The practicalities of researching sexuality

Although research into the causes and signs of homosexuality has not yet been abandoned, researchers are increasingly following very different lines of enquiry. Demand is growing in the health and social care professions, both from service users and practitioners, for research data that can be used to drive positive developments in sexuality-related policy and practice. This demand, in combination with increasing social tolerance, has led to an opening up of this field of research. However, researchers into sexuality still find that they face particular problems.

Until recently it was almost impossible for those working in health and social care to carry out research into lesbian or gay issues. Interest in homosexuality tends to carry with it a stigma by association, the assumption being that you would not be interested in those people unless you yourself were 'like that' (Plummer 1981). Anyone suspected of being gay risked losing their friends, their professional credibility or even their job. Such experiences continue to be reported in the literature (see, for example, Rule 1985; Warland 1992; Jackson 1998), but they are now less common. However, as one recent account demonstrates, researchers are still faced with uncooperative or dismissive attitudes:

> a 'flagship' GUM service, . . . which had initially agreed to participate in my research, declined at the last moment to do so (after full ethics committee approval had been granted), on the grounds that it was not possible to find a member of clinic staff willing to take named responsibility for liaising with a study on lesbian sexual health. [. . .] Secondly, when I attempted to approach the director of an alternative clinic, who was known for her innovatory (published) views on sexual health service provision for women, I was rebuffed on the grounds that the clinic 'doesn't see any lesbians.'
>
> (Farquhar 1999: 81)

The guiding principle of most research up to the 1970s was that homosexuality was a pathological condition. This made it difficult for lesbian and gay service users to participate in research, and also for researchers to gain the trust necessary for meaningful collaboration (Farquhar 1999; Institute of Medicine 1999). Above all, those who agree to be the subjects/participants in such research continue to put themselves at risk. For a significant number of people, the risks of coming out remain serious.

Making research possible: feminism and AIDS

There has been a gradual liberalisation of sexual mores in twentieth-century Western culture, but specific social and political factors also acted as catalysts for research into homosexuality. The Women's Liberation Movement (WLM) saw a dramatic resurgence of activity in the 1960s, the so-called 'Second Wave' of feminism (nineteenth-century campaigns for suffrage and social equality being the First Wave). The WLM was generally hostile to lesbians (Abbott and Love 1985; Wilton 1995), and feminist health activists to this day are criticised for ignoring lesbian issues (Wilton 1996; Farquhar 1999). Nevertheless, feminist political theory and activism, in the context of a burgeoning women's health movement, undoubtedly did much to lay the foundations for research and activism in lesbian health.

For gay men the problems were different. For two decades, lesbians fought alongside other women in battles over reproductive health, abortion rights, choice in childbirth, mental health, breast and cervical cancer and other important issues where sexism was a significant factor. During that period, health issues remained a low priority for gay men. All that changed when the early years of the AIDS pandemic in the US and Europe forced health issues to the front of gay men's minds. Although AIDS is still the number one research priority in gay men's health, research funded in response to the epidemic revealed more general failures in knowledge, attitudes and practices amongst health and social care professionals working with this group (Coxon 1988; Davies *et al.* 1990, 1993; Kayal 1993).

As well as the WLM and the AIDS emergency, more general social shifts towards decriminalisation, greater tolerance and a degree of support for equality have led to increased opportunities for researchers. Funding bodies can now be persuaded that research into lesbian and gay issues is worthwhile, and institutional employers such as the NHS, local authority social services departments and universities are more likely to support those engaged in such work. Things have improved almost beyond recognition since the days when showing an interest in lesbian or gay issues would get you the sack (Rule 1985).

Existing research and its findings

Most research into lesbian and gay experiences of health and social care comes from the United States. Outwith the specialisms associated with AIDS, most has been located in nursing, with gradually increasing contributions from midwifery, social work and youth work. Given the organisation and delivery of healthcare within the US, it is perhaps not surprising that psychotherapy, counselling and substance abuse treatment programmes have also paid significant attention to the needs of their lesbian and gay clients.

In Britain, nursing seems to have taken the lead, with the Royal College of Nursing setting up a working party on lesbian and gay nursing issues.

The survey research that they carried out led to much discussion in the nursing press, and eventually resulted in the publication of a formal RCN Statement, *The Nursing Care of Lesbians and Gay Men* (Royal College of Nursing 1994) (see Appendix).

The need for interprofessional collaboration

The greater proportion of research into lesbian and gay issues in health and social care is carried out by concerned professionals, most of whom are themselves lesbian or gay (Farquhar 1999). Investigative methods and epistemologies are therefore shaped by the research traditions and protocols of the different professions within health and social care, and findings tend to be fairly narrowly disseminated via the practice literature. This impedes the accumulation of a rigorous knowledge base and the development of effective policies and practices *across* health and social care, since hard-pressed staff do not have the time or energy to read widely outside their own professional journals. A ground-breaking article in *The Nursing Times* is unlikely to be of much use to a social worker or physiotherapist. A certain amount of reinventing the wheel inevitably results, although this problem is not confined to sexualities research.

The drive towards professionalisation, the question of accountability and increasing concern about bad practice have led to a new emphasis, particularly in nursing (Thompson 1995), on evidence-based practice and the relexive practitioner. The aim is to produce not just a 'knowledgeable doer', but one who is able to respond to new information – including that which comes from reflecting on personal practice – with appropriate changes. In order to develop the 'research' that must underpin practice and the 'knowledge' that supports the individual practitioner, it is necessary to draw on any and all available literature, in whatever professional context it may be found. What follows is a summary of research into the experiences of lesbian, gay and bisexual users of health and social care services, trawled from the academic and practice literature of many sources: social work, nursing, youth and community work, lesbian and gay studies, counselling and education.

A familiar story

A full review of this literature would itself require a substantial book. However, for reasons which by now are familiar, research articles may be hard to track down; many are in highly specialised publications such as the *Journal of Homosexuality* or the *Journal of Gay and Lesbian Social Services*, which may not be available in some libraries. Some are only available in the form of unpublished postgraduate dissertations or conference papers, whilst others may be found in relatively ephemeral sources such as the gay press. Below are some key findings of recent research into lesbian and gay health and social care experiences in the US and Britain.

- Many health and social care professionals, including general practitioners and clinical specialists, are ill-informed about lesbian and gay health issues. For example, many GPs wrongly believe that lesbians do not need cervical smears.
- Many health and social care professionals (the majority of respondants in some surveys) hold ill-informed and prejudicial beliefs about lesbian and gay people and their lifestyles.
- A significant proportion of lesbians and gay men who make their sexual orientation known to health and social care staff experience poor treatment, hostility or abuse in consequences.
- Education and training about lesbian and gay issues is absent or inadequate throughout the health and social care professional field. Only in specialist areas such as HIV/AIDS are such issues fully addressed. This perpetuates a degree of ignorance which is, in some cases, quite startling.
- There is increasing concern that medical knowledge is *itself* likely to perpetuate negative attitudes; studies have found negative images of homosexuality or 'subtle' homophobia and heterosexism in health-care literature, including textbooks.
- The statutory powers of health and social services continue to be used in ways that discriminate against lesbians and gay men.
- A significant number of lesbian and gay service users feel too unsafe to come out to doctors and other health and social care professionals. In consequence, many delay seeking treatment, or may seek advice only from sympathetic complementary practitioners, or even from untrained friends.

(These findings are summarised from: Hidalgo *et al.* 1985; Shernoff and Scott 1988; Schwanberg 1990; Cossis Brown 1992; Whatley 1992; Stern 1993; McClure and Vespry 1994; Das 1996; Hardman 1996; Muir-Mackenzie and Orme 1996; Peterson 1996; Sheffield Health 1996; Stewart 1997; Wilton and Hall 1998; Farquhar 1999; Mugglestone 1999).

Summarising his own review of the health-care literature, Schwartz (1993: 31) concludes that 'Blatant homophobia, heterosexism, inadequate knowledge and discrimination within the health care system are common experiences'. Such findings give serious cause for concern.

One survey of attitudes held by nursing students towards lesbians uncovered powerful feelings of disgust and revulsion. Comments included: 'They are sick . . . they are not normal human beings. They try to turn young, normal people into lesbians with their gay marches,' 'they are ugly women who can't get dates with men' and 'normal human beings [can] contract lesbianism like a contagious disease' (Eliason and Randall 1991: 46–47). One UK study (Rose 1993) found that more than a quarter of a sample of nurses interviewed had witnessed colleagues refusing to give care to a homosexual patient, whilst another (Hoolaghan *et al.* 1993) found that GPs felt less able to address sexual issues with lesbians than with any other group.

Other studies have shown, not surprisingly, that being nursed by people with such prejudicial attitudes is not only unpleasant, but may also be unsafe (Darty and Potter 1984; Savage 1987). Several researchers (Lyon

Martin Women's Health Services 1993; Stevens 1993; Trippet and Bain 1993; Pollinger Haas 1994) find evidence that disclosure of sexual orientation in health care environments 'constitutes a health risk in and of itself; causing repeated stress' (Farquhar 1999: 92). Such stress is magnified when lack of continuity of care forces patients and service users to come out repeatedly.

Those whose work requires/enables them to develop a caring relationship with patients/clients are well placed to understand the professional requirement for compassion and respect. Yet the attitudes of those whose face-to-face contact with service users is minimal – including radiographers, pharmacists and receptionists – may be equally significant, as this account from a hospital social worker makes clear:

> Marc, a client with AIDS, went to the hospital pharmacy to pick up his AZT ... the pharmacist told him that queers and faggots who have AIDS need to sit in an isolated section of the waiting room ...
>   (Schwartz 1993: 27)

Although this is perhaps an extreme example, it is far from being an isolated incident. There are similar accounts from other lesbian or gay service users who found themselves on the receiving end of insulting or abusive comments (James *et al.* 1994; Annesley 1995; Dockery 1996; Sheffield Health 1996; Hardman 1997; Harwood 1998; Mugglestone 1999). If concepts such as continuity of care or inter-agency working are at all meaningful, all staff – even those whose contact with users is minimal – must recognise that casual homophobia of this kind has the potential to hurt or harm.

The conclusions of over two decades of research are, sadly, unambiguous. Lesbians and gay men who use health and social care services are accustomed to being treated with contempt, hostility and neglect. Of course, attitudes are starting to change. However, even the most recent research indicates continuing and serious failures in care. These failures range from obvious discomfort, rudeness or hostility on the part of staff to clear instances where homophobia has led to poor quality care:

> '... a doctor thought I was ill *because* of my sexuality. In fact, it was chronic fatigue syndrome.'

> 'My partner was not allowed to be with me because she wasn't family or husband! after an accident I had.'

> 'One male doctor in the Clinic ... was clearly *not* comfortable carrying out a full sexual health check on a gay man.'

> 'I asked my GP whether, as someone who hadn't had sex with a man, I needed a cervical smear. *She* didn't know and didn't make much effort to find out.'
>   (Wilton and Hall 1998)

It would be misleading to suggest that such attitudes are expressed by *all* health and social care staff, or that all lesbian and gay service users have bad experiences all the time. Many health and social care professionals are themselves lesbian or gay, and many others clearly do their best to offer respectful and considerate care. Where good quality care is offered without undue fuss it is deeply appreciated:

> 'Although it was difficult at first to be out to my GP he has been very accepting and supportive, as have other members of the practice.'

> 'When I was unwell, my GP was positive about my lesbian partner – she assumed my partner would be supportive to me.'

> 'Community midwives delivered both children at home with me and my partner. They were *BRILLIANT.*'
>
> (Wilton and Hall 1998)

Staff who treat lesbian and gay service users well deserve respect and recognition for their efforts. However, until professional training universally supports good practice in this area, the quality of care received by lesbians and gay men remains a lottery.

Implications for practice

The practicalities of integrating research, theory and practice are a continuing problem for the caring professions (Thompson 1995). In the field of sexuality where, as we have learned, information may be located in unfamiliar disciplines, hidden in the 'grey' literature or otherwise inaccessible, existing problems are magnified. This section critically evaluates the kinds of information currently available and presents a case study demonstrating that improvements in service delivery may require staff to take steps normally regarded as outside their professional boundaries. This suggests that 'research' must be reconceptualised to encompass learning and information-gathering strategies *additional to* the formal techniques of academic inquiry.

Learning from past mistakes: a case study

Providing *effective* services to lesbians and gay men may require proactive interventions far wider than non-discriminatory treatment, as this case history from the American social work literature suggests.

> Mary and Carol had been partners for ten years, and taken formal steps to safeguard their mutual interests. They shared a home and a bank account and had even borrowed money to secure a burial site together.

> Carol received lengthy periods of medical treatment for serious conditions, and at all times the hospital staff respected their wishes to have Mary recognised as next of kin. When warned her partner was dying, Mary told Carol's long-estranged birth family of her critical condition. Carol's mother promptly took her daughter out of hospital and back to the family home, making it clear that Mary was not welcome. Mary then discovered that the shared bank account had been closed, leaving her unable to access her money.
>
> Mary was refused all contact with Carol, who died alone. Her family, ignoring her wishes, held a Catholic funeral and scattered her ashes on her father's grave. Mary was forced to sell their home. She was also obliged to continue paying off the loan for the burial site the two women had chosen. Most devastating of all was the terrible grief of knowing that her partner had died alone (Connolly 1996).
>
> The health care staff and social workers involved in Carol's care fulfilled their professional responsibilities and treated Carol and Mary with respect. However, had any member of the team involved in Carol's care been properly trained in the issues confronting lesbians and gay men with terminal illnesses, they might have done more to encourage Carol to make a will, or to establish Mary's status legally, and might have thought to discuss with both Mary and Carol the questions raised by Carol's estrangement from her birth family. As Connolly concludes (1996: 85), 'the most important lesson of this case study is that, to prevent this from happening again, the health and social service providers have to go beyond their normal routines and responsibilities.' Yet few resources exist to support or inform staff in such demanding circumstances.

The situation is, of course, different in the UK. The Royal College of Nursing has found that, 'some nurses refuse to acknowledge the status of a same-sex partner, denying visiting rights and access to information', but points out that '[t]here is often no legal basis for these actions and they may also be unprofessional' (Royal College of Nursing 1998). In fact, the concept of next-of-kin status has very limited legal meaning, and offers no justification for refusing to recognise the wishes of a lesbian or gay service user with regard to the status of their partner. The Mental Health Act and the Children Act do make specific provisions and, in such cases, appropriate guidance should be sought.

The information problem

The inability of staff to meet the needs of lesbian or gay service users stems in part from major failures in basic and post-basic training and education (Cossis Brown 1992; Stevens 1993; Das 1996; Sheffield Health 1996; Farquhar 1999). Little attention is paid to questions of sexuality in training, and often no time at all is allocated to lesbian and gay issues (L. Jones 1994). The picture is no less bleak if we turn to those areas of the curriculum intended to cover such questions – sociology and psychology.

To take sociology as a 'case study'; an examination of some of the most popular textbooks used to teach social science in health and social care (Armstrong 1989; Baggott 1994; L. Jones 1994; Moon and Gillespie 1995; Nettleton 1995; Annandale 1998) reveals an almost complete disregard for sexuality and silence on the subject of homosexuality. Yet these introductory texts typically discuss issues such as doctor–patient interaction, stigma, medicalisation, gender roles, social exclusion, self-help groups and critiques of medical practice (such as anti-racism and feminism). Lesbian and gay issues are directly relevant to these questions, and there is a strong argument that some of them may not be adequately theorised *without* reference to sexuality (Wilton 1995; Farquhar 1999).

This reluctance to recognise the significance of sexuality as a social variable is self-perpetuating. Students depending on such textbooks for information about the sociology of health, illness and medicine are left with the impression that sexuality is simply not an issue. This is a failure of C. Wright Mills's famous 'sociological imagination' but also, more disturbingly, contributes to the discursive construction of heterosexuality as the unproblematic norm, which causes such harm in the practice of health and social care. Those working in the field have a continuing struggle to find adequate sources of evidence to underpin innovative practice developments in this neglected area.

The existence of a women's health movement underpinned by feminist theory has offered a useful framework for innovations in lesbian health. However, neither the feminist literature on health nor feminist research are exempt from the charge of heterosexism. Although there are honourable exceptions, the approach taken by the recently published *Pennell Report*, a well-funded literature review on older women's health, is more typical. The authors write: 'we have not . . . explored the healthcare needs and experiences of lesbians. We have, in the main, referred to information about the population generally' (Pennell Initiative 1998: 5). Publishing in 1998, the authors – professional researchers – had easy access to a growing literature on lesbian health. Think back to the earlier discussion of health promotion as a discourse; what effect do you think it might have for a major research report to ignore lesbians in this way, and to refer to 'the population generally' as a group from which lesbians are *excluded*?

From the community or in the community?

Many innovations in lesbian and gay health and social care have grown out of community activism. Such activism has taken place across the traditional practitioner–client divide. As it has become less risky to be 'out' at work, lesbians, gay men and bisexuals working in health and social care have initiated various schemes in support of anti-discriminatory practice. Some have set up working parties or support groups, either within the framework of a union or professional body (as in the case of NALGO or the Royal College of Nursing's Lesbian and Gay Working Party) or separately (for example, the National Organisation of Lesbian and Gay Youth and Community Workers).

Motivated in part by the post-Stonewall mood of defiance and partly by the growth of a consumerist model of citizenship, service users have also fought for change. They have established self-help groups, campaigning organisations and telephone helplines. Sometimes these services are entirely separate from the statutory sector – as is the case for local lesbian and gay telephone helplines. Others represent a mix of voluntary and statutory, or may draw on a combination of professional and user involvement. A good example of the 'mixed economy' approach may be seen in the lesbian sexual health clinics or drop-in centres now to be found in several cities in Britian. Such centres have a close relationship to the wider women's health movement, and have a long history. The first, at St Mark's Clinic in New York, was established in 1973 (Vida 1978). In Britain, the Audre Lorde and Sandra Bernhardt Clinics in London hospitals, set up by a lesbian GUM specialist, were swiftly followed by others in Oxford and Glasgow (Wilton 1998).

Community expertise: AIDS services

One of the most extraordinary examples of good practice springing from the gay community itself has been its response to the HIV pandemic. Neglected by those supposedly responsible for protecting public health, this marginalised group was able to respond in a way which appears, in retrospect, nothing short of heroic. As a result of official indifference, *all* the money for AIDS research in the early years of the epidemic came from fund raising in the gay community (Shilts 1987; Kayal 1993; Wilton 1997a). It was gay men, not doctors, who first reached the conclusion that the new syndrome was likely to be caused by a transmissible organism (Patton 1985; Kayal 1993). It was also gay men who invented safe sex, both the term and the practice, despite the fact that many gay men had never even seen a condom.

AIDS service organisations, such as Gay Men's Health Crisis in New York or the Terrence Higgins Trust in Britain, grew out of lesbian and gay community activism, but were from the start open to anyone, gay or straight, who needed them. Lesbians took responsibility for developing and distributing safer sex information to women, worked on AIDS helplines, joined in the fund-raising and political activism, and worked as carers, buddies and counsellors (Patton 1985; Richardson 1994). In the US, groups of lesbians calling themselves 'blood sisters' donated blood so that enough would be available to meet the needs of gay men with AIDS.

Whilst all this exemplary good citizenship was going on, governments, the press, the media and the Christian right kept up a constant barrage of abuse against the community (Altman 1986; Kramer 1990; Kayal 1993). Nor were all the problems coming from outside; many gay men thought AIDS was yet another excuse to police their sex lives, while some lesbians were unwilling to put energy into helping gay men who had, after all, never shown much interest in lesbian health issues. Nevertheless, it is widely acknowledged that the infrastructure of AIDS service work that exists in the Western world today originated in the lesbian and gay community.

Some of these initiatives have become major institutions; groups such as the Terrence Higgins Trust have established themselves as the primary location of expertise as well as support. The best example is Gay Men's Health Crisis in New York. This voluntary organisation, set up in the earliest days of the AIDS epidemic, is now the largest specialist AIDS organisation in the world and the level of expertise developed by their volunteers has led to it becoming recognised as one of the best sources of clinical information about HIV disease and therapeutic developments. The GMFA newsletter, *Treatment Issues*, is the bible of hundreds of clinical practitioners in the field, as well as thousands of individuals living with HIV.

Perhaps the greatest achievement has been the extent to which gay men have succeeded in making safer sex an integral part of gay identity. They have developed a forthright and imaginative approach which, whilst recognising the complexity of people's sexual feelings and behaviours, presents safer sex as a necessary element in caring relationships, in community responsibility and in gay identity itself. Safer sex materials developed by gay activists retain a close relationship with the communities that they target. Thus, they are able to respond swiftly to new developments and to offer a range of materials that reflect the diversity within the gay subculture (Wilton 1997a). Strenuous attempts have been made to reach out to the silent thousands of men who continue to think of themselves as heterosexual, despite having casual sex with other men. A health education campaign of this intensity, variety and effectiveness has never been seen before, let alone in the context of the severe discrimination faced by the gay community.

However, there are drawbacks to this dependence on community energy and expertise. As AIDS activist Tony Whitehead warns (1993: 107), the 'well-intentioned but perhaps misguided complicity between charity and the statutory sector . . . has allowed the latter consistently to avoid the fundamental issues and demands raised by the British epidemic.' In an astute analysis of the establishment response to AIDS, Whitehead (1993: 108) suggests that:

> the Government wanted to get as much money from the community as it possibly could in order to reduce its own level of funding. It was also clear that it wanted to keep itself as far away as possible from any closely targeted education towards gay men and drug users.

Lesbian sexual health clinics

Similar criticisms could be made of lesbian sexual health clinics. Such initiatives are only needed because failures in existing services make them useless to most lesbians (Evans and Farquhar 1995; Farquhar 1999). Although there has been an enormously enthusiastic response to the lesbian clinics, they do present a dilemma. Where they are situated in existing hospital GUM departments, they may offer valuable learning opportunities for NHS staff. However, when they are situated in the local community, as is the case in Glasgow (Ilett 1995), they often depend on the dedication of volunteers. Critics point out that this may actually discourage managers from making needful improvements in statutory services.

The question of how to make the best use of community expertise, energy and commitment, without allowing the statutory services to evade their responsibilities, is a difficult one. It is not confined to lesbian and gay communities, but is especially acute for them, given their long history of neglect by the statutory agencies. This difficult balance makes it still more important that health and social care practitioners take steps to facilitate whatever improvements are needed in their own area of service provision.

Practical elements of good practice

It is helpful to conclude this survey of research findings with some pointers towards elements of good practice. From existing studies it is clear that good practice depends on practitioners who are both informed and self-critical, working in environments that are positively welcoming to users and staff regardless of sexual orientation.

Self-education

The traditional model of all-knowing expert dispensing advice to ignorant lay people no longer underpins health and social care to the extent that it once did. Just as realisation slowly dawned in health and social care that the best experts on minority ethnic communities were members of those communities themselves, it is starting to be recognised that the best experts on what it means to be lesbian, gay or bisexual may not be geneticists, endocrinologists, priests, rabbis, psychiatrists or even sociologists, but gay people themselves.

However this can result in additional stress for service users. Lesbians and gay men frequently complain that they are obliged to act as informal health and social care trainers, in a necessary effort to counteract the ignorance and misinformation of those caring for them (Hidalgo et al. 1985; Stern 1993; Davies and Neal 1996; Sheffield Health 1996; Wilton and Hall 1998; Farquhar 1999).

An additional problem for the health and social care professional who depends on the goodwill of 'out' clients/patients for information is that it is unlikely that most clients or patients will *be* 'out' in a health or social care context. Concealing one's sexual orientation is often a necessary coping strategy, and there is evidence that this may be especially true of Black or other minority ethnic service users (Cossis Brown 1992; Hidalgo 1995).

This produces a dilemma. These coping strategies, necessary though they are, may mask need. The first element of good practice must therefore be for the practitioner to take responsibility for learning about the lives of lesbians and gay men, about the issues that may arise in a practice situation, and about strategies for proactively supporting lesbian, gay and bisexual service users.

Attitudinal reflexivity

Research also indicates that knowledge on its own is not enough. Prejudice against lesbian and gay people is a deeply-woven strand in Western societies and this makes it hard for individuals, however committed they may be, to erase its trace from their own unconscious behaviours, such as body language. Any negative reactions of staff may be clearly perceived by the client despite attempts at concealment. One survey of lesbian users of mental health services found that:

> A few women reported having attended closely to their clinical psychologist's verbal and nonverbal responses in order to gauge the reaction that their disclosure [of sexuality] engendered. For example, one said 'She actually looked shocked and she shut up . . . and she just went, moved slightly backwards, yes, and just an involuntary thing as she stopped talking, a very slight lean back and immediately carried on talking to me as if she hadn't been shocked but she was because I could tell by her body language'.
>
> (Annesley 1995: 7)

Another lesbian, interviewed about her experiences with cervical smear services reported that she:

> made the mistake of coming out to the practice nurse when she was getting ready to take a smear . . . I heard this loud 'Clang!' She'd dropped the speculum on the floor. She was not offensive to me, but she was obviously shocked and embarrassed.
>
> (Wilton 1997b: 208)

Lesbians and gay men are highly aware of such signals. The second requirement of good practice is therefore that practitioners should continue to reflect on their own attitudes and beliefs. This is a difficult process, and one which should not be confused with a superficial 'politically correct' approach. At every point in this book it has been clear that heterosexism and homophobia are powerful social forces, not minor personal failings (Kitzinger 1987).

Respondents to some surveys suggest, and the wider literature confirms, that personal familiarity with lesbian and gay lives and communities is the best predictor of relaxed attitudes and lack of bias (Clark 1987; Pharr 1988; Sheffield Health 1996). Of course, it is not always easy to acquire 'personal familiarity', but there is ample material available to teach and inform about gay lives and communities. Autobiographies, collections of coming out stories, gay cartoon collections and gay magazines all offer material that is both informative and easy to read (see the 'Resources' section at the end of this chapter).

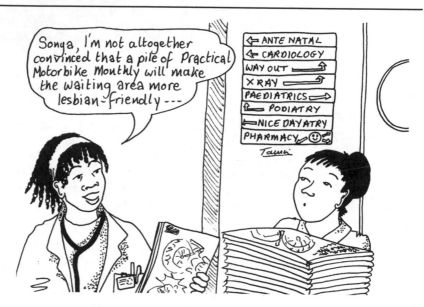

Creating a safe environment

Even the most conscientious individual is able to exercise only a limited influence in their professional environment, and that environment matters a lot. Researchers have found that male-dominated work places have the effect of excluding women by displays of pornography or pictures of sports cars or by employing metaphors taken from football or cricket in the board room (Cockburn 1985, 1991). Similarly, most public environments are resolutely, albeit unconsciously, heterosexist. Against this background, it does not take much effort to give a welcoming signal to lesbians and gay men. One recent survey found that 'lesbians wanted to see openly lesbian-friendly services which would require . . . the displaying of relevant leaflets and posters by health care establishments' (Sheffield Health 1996: 38). This suggests that the third element in good practice might well be to take whatever steps are possible to make your work environment more gay-friendly.

Such steps need not be difficult and will not involve cost. The local gay switchboard almost certainly prints cards advertising its services and hours of opening. Pin these to the notice-board in your clinic, day-care centre or coffee bar, and you are signalling your recognition that not all service users are heterosexual. Scatter a few magazines around the waiting area. *Diva*, for example, is a glossy lesbian magazine, which would not look out of place in a pile of *Cosmopolitan* or *Vogue*, and many lesbian and gay communities produce local newsletters or magazines. An appeal for back issues means that you will not even have to pay for them.

A degree of sensitivity is required, however! Some gay men's magazines, such as *Gay Times*, have to serve the function of a whole range of publications in the heterosexual mainstream. Thus, although they contain much useful information, they may also include explicit advertisements for services such as telephone sex lines or dating services, and you may feel that leaving them in the waiting area is inappropriate.

Radiographers often stick calming pictures to the ceiling above X-ray machines and other diagnostic equipment; physiotherapy gymnasia and exercise suites tend to have images of happy people, resolutely exercising away. It is not difficult to find lesbian or gay images to add to the display. Such images need not be explicit, a picture of Justin Fashanu or Martina Navratilova might serve the purpose. There are images – such as a shot from the Gay Games or a photograph of a gay football team – which would be 'read' as gay friendly by a lesbian or gay client/patient, but which would pass unnoticed by others. Heterosexuals may be able to call on the insider knowledge of lesbian and gay colleagues to track down such images.

Updating and referral skills

A career in health or social care means working extremely hard at a demanding job with little spare time. Nobody could ever acquire all the knowledge necessary to respond effectively to every possible scenario where sexuality becomes an issue. The fourth demand of good practice is therefore that practitioners update their own information – by reading the professional literature and the gay press – but also that they make themselves aware of other sources of information to which they may refer their clients/patients for additional support. Every health and social care professional, for example, should know the number of their local lesbian and gay switchboard, and should have some idea of where to get information about lesbian and gay issues if and when the need arises.

Professional and institutional support

All these elements of good practice involve individual practitioners. As such, they may expose those practitioners to various kinds of risk in the exercise of their professional obligations. The continued widespread failure to recognise homophobia as an unacceptable form of discrimination means that any attempts at change may meet with negative reactions from colleagues, managers, heterosexual service users or even – and this is probably the worst nightmare of every social services or healthcare trust director – the press or media. This is why good practice in this area also requires interventions at the level of policy.

An equal opportunities policy, which includes sexual orientation, offers valuable protection to staff and service users. It is equally important that unions and professional bodies recognise the significance of sexuality in health and social care, and have policies supporting anti-homophobic practice. Such policies are especially necessary in the education and training of health and social care professionals, and should be as explicit as possible. For example, the RCN statement on *The Nursing Care of Lesbians and Gay Men* (see Appendix) includes a paragraph outlining the responsibility of nurse tutors to design pre- and post-registration courses about lesbian and gay issues in nursing. This offers much more substantial support than the requirement of the Central Council for Education and Training in Social Work (CCETSW) that 'candidates for the Diploma in Social Work must demonstrate their competence in non-discriminatory and non-oppressive social work practice' (Cossis Brown 1992: 201). Of course, unions, work places and professional bodies seldom make or change policies without prompting, so this final element of good practice makes it the responsibility of practitioners to lobby for change where necessary.

In summary, the principles of good practice relating to sexuality in health and social care are:

1 Practitioners should take responsibility for learning about the lives of lesbians, gay men and bisexuals, about the issues which may arise in their professional practice, and about strategies for proactively protecting the interests of this user group.
2 Practitioners should examine their own attitudes towards, and beliefs about, sexualities that differ from their own, in line with the requirements of reflexive practice.
3 All possible steps should be taken to make health and social care environments welcoming to lesbian, gay and bisexual service users.
4 Practitioners should keep themselves informed of changing issues affecting this user group, and should make themselves aware of local sources of advice, information and support.
5 Equal opportunities policies should make explicit reference to sexual orientation, as should the written standards of professional bodies. Practitioners should take whatever steps are necessary to ensure that this is the case, in their own interests and that of their clients.

Conclusion

The health and social care professions have a troubled history in relation to their lesbian and gay service users. Much suffering has been caused, sometimes with malicious intent but often out of a misplaced desire to do good. By medicalising sexuality, medicine has been particularly complicit in the policing of sexual and intimate behaviours in society more widely. Social work and youth work, on the other hand, have a history of complicity with wider projects of social control involving the regulation of families and the promotion of heterosexist familial ideologies. It is important to acknowledge this history and to understand its implications for current practice and for the relationship between health care, social care and lesbian and gay service users.

Social and cultural changes, including the post-Stonewall lesbian and gay liberation movement, the women's movement and the AIDS crisis, have contributed to a growing liberalisation of attitudes towards homosexuality. This has been reflected in health and social care, as practitioners are able to be more open about their sexuality and to develop practice initiatives in support of their lesbian and gay clientele. This has been paralleled by activism in the community, and the establishment of alternative community services. There has also been an increase in research activity, and much is now known about the specific needs of lesbian and gay service users.

In short, the health and social care professions are witnessing a new era, with exciting potential for research, development and practice. Although much remains to be done, there is increasing evidence of determination to remedy the mistakes of the past. Given what we are starting to learn about the consequences of sexual orientation for health and well-being, and about the individual and social disbenefits of social exclusion and discrimination, it is starting to become clear that people of *all* sexualities stand to gain from innovations in research and practice.

Far from needing 'special treatment', lesbian, gay and bisexual service users share fundamental human needs, which need to be dealt with in appropriate ways. Moreover, as we have seen, failing to recognise the significance of sexuality may have unhelpful consequences for heterosexual service users as much as for those who are lesbian, gay or bisexual. In the long run, health and welfare provision which is underpinned by more sophisticated understandings of human sexual diversity, and premised on a more inclusive account of human rights and human need, will be better for all of us.

---

exercise

What follows is a real life case study taken from the caseload of a hospital social worker. Read it through carefully, then answer the questions which follow.

Evan was dying of AIDS when he was hospitalized by his lover, Bruce. The latter notified Evan's family who appeared the next day. Within a few minutes of their arrival, Bruce was informed by the attending physician that he could no longer stay with Evan and that he, the doctor, would follow whatever instructions the family gave him regarding maintaining Bruce's life. The family had informed the doctor that Bruce had seduced Evan into the deviant lifestyle of homosexuality and that Bruce should be banned from visiting Evan. Bruce was not permitted to say goodbye to his partner, nor was he part of the funeral.

(Taken from Schwartz 1993: 29–30)

1 How could this situation have been prevented?

2 What steps could Bruce have taken to ensure that he was able to remain with his lover?

3 Whose responsibility is it to make sure Bruce and Evan know their rights and take the appropriate steps to protect them?

4 What do you think of the doctor's behaviour? Was he right? To what extent is he bound by the law in this case?

5 What similar circumstances might arise in your own practice area? What could you, personally, do to help in this situation? What might you do beforehand to *prevent* such a situation?

6 What difference do you think it would make if either or both partners were Muslim? Or Jewish?

7 Do you know what sources of legal advice or other support are available to help Bruce and Evan? Could you put them in touch with the appropriate services?

8 If this case history has revealed gaps in your knowledge or your practice, how do you intend to rectify this? If it has revealed particular strengths, how may you best put these to good use?

Resources

This section is more substantial than in previous chapters, since it is intended to support the self-education process that underpins the development of good practice for individual practitioners in health and social care.

History

Blasius, M. and Phelan, S. (1997) *We Are Everywhere: A Historical Sourcebook of Gay and Lesbian Politics*. London: Routledge.

Grau, G. (1993) *Hidden Holocaust? Gay and Lesbian Persecution in Germany 1933–45*. London: Cassell.

Hamer, E. (1996) *Britannia's Glory: A History of Twentieth-Century Lesbians*. London: Cassell.

Healey, E. and Mason, A. (eds) *Stonewall 25: The Making of the Lesbian and Gay Community in Britain*. London: Virago.

Miller, N. (1995) *Out of the Past: Gay and Lesbian History from 1869 to the Present*. New York: Vintage Books.

Autobiography

Collected stories

Hall-Carpenter Archives Lesbian Oral History Group (1989) *Inventing Ourselves: Lesbian Life Stories*. London: Routledge.

Holmes, S. (ed.) (1988) *Testimonies: A Collection of Lesbian Coming Out Stories*. Boston: Alyson Books.

National Lesbian and Gay Survey (1992) *What a Lesbian Looks Like: Writings by Lesbians on Their Lives and Lifestyles*. London: Routledge.

National Lesbian and Gay Survey (1993) *Proust, Cole Porter, Michaelangelo, Marc Almond and Me: Writings by Gay Men on Their Lives and Lifestyles*. London: Routledge.

Neild, S. and Pearson, R. (eds) (1992) *Women Like Us* (the stories of older lesbians). London: The Women's Press.

Umans, M. (1988) *Like Coming Home: Coming-Out Letters*. Austin, TX: Banned Books.

Individual autobiographies

Crisp, Q. (1968) *The Naked Civil Servant*. London: Collins.

Grey, A. (1997) *Speaking Out: Sex, Law, Politics and Society 1954–1995*. London: Cassell.

Lorde, A. (1982) *Zami: A New Spelling of My Name*. London: Sheba.

Manning, R. (1987) *A Corridor of Mirrors*. London: The Women's Press.

White, E. (1982) *A Boy's Own Story*. London: Picador.

Professional and practice issues

Davies, D. and Neal, C. (eds) (1996) *Pink Therapy: A Guide for Counsellors and Therapists Working with Lesbian, Gay and Bisexual Clients*. Buckingham: Open University Press.

Epstein, D. (ed.) (1994) *Challenging Lesbian and Gay Inequalities in Education*. Buckingham: Open University Press.

Gruskin, E.P. (1999) *Treating Lesbians and Bisexual Women: Challenges and Strategies for Health Professionals*. Thousand Oaks, CA: Sage.

Hidalgo, H. (1995) *Lesbians of Colour: Social and Human Services*. New York: Haworth Press.

Hidalgo, H., Peterson, T. and Woodman, N.J. (eds) (1985) *Lesbian and Gay Issues: A Resource Manual for Social Workers*. Washington, DC: National Association of Social Workers.

Institute of Medicine (1999) *Lesbian Health: Current Assessment and Directions for the Future*. Washington: National Academy Press.

Savage, J. (1987) *Nurses, Gender and Sexuality*. London: Heinemann.

Shakespeare, T., Gillespie-Sells, K. and Davies, D. (eds) (1996) *The Sexual Politics of Disability*. London: Cassell.

Whitlock, K. (1988) *Bridges of Respect: Creating Support for Lesbian and Gay Youth*. Philadelphia: The American Friends Service Committee.

Wilton, T. (1998) *Good For You: A Handbook on Lesbian Health and Wellbeing*. London: Cassell.

Lesbian Health Matters: a Training Video is available from London Lesbians in Health Care, c/o The Wheel, Wild Court, off Kingsway, London WC2B 4AU.

Exploring different avenues

Ali, T. (1996) *We Are Family: Testimonies of Lesbian and Gay Parents*. London: Cassell.

Griffin, K. and Mulholland, L. (eds) (1997) *Lesbian Motherhood in Europe*. London: Cassell.

Hamilton, A. and Guthries, M. (1997) *The Lesbian and Gay Rights Handbook*. London: Cassell.

Reinfelder, M. (ed.) (1995) *Amazon to Zami: Towards a Global Lesbian Feminism*. London: Cassell.

Stuart, E. (1992) *Daring to Speak Love's Name: A Gay and Lesbian Prayer Book*. London: Hamish Hamilton.

Turner, M. (1998) *Through the Minefields: Implementing Lesbian and Gay Equal Opportunities Policies in Local Government, Education Establishments, Charities and Non-Statutory Agencies Through Training*. London: Cassell.

Exploring lesbian and gay studies

Abelove, H., Barale, M.A. and Halperin, D. (eds) (1993) *The Lesbian and Gay Studies Reader*. London: Routledge.

Horne, P. and Lewis, R. (eds) (1996) *Outlooks: Lesbian and Gay Sexualities and Visual Cultures*. London: Routledge.

Nardi, P. and Schneider, B. (eds) (1998) *Social Perspectives in Lesbian and Gay Studies: a Reader*. London: Routledge.

Plummer, K. (ed.) (1992) *Modern Homosexualities: Fragments of the Lesbian and Gay Experience*. London: Routledge.

Wilton, T. (1995) *Lesbian Studies: Setting an Agenda*. London: Routledge.

Journals

Sexualities
GLQ: A Journal of Lesbian and Gay Studies

Sources of information

For books and magazines (mail order service):

Gay's The Word Bookshop, 66 Marchmont Street, London WC1N 1AB Tel: 020 7278 7654

London Lesbian and Gay Switchboard: 020 7837 7324

London Lesbian Line: 020 7251 6911

Gay and Lesbian Legal Advice: BM GLAD, London WC1N 3XX

Lesbian Information Service: PO Box 194, Leicester LE1 9HP

Stonewall: 16 Clerkenwell Close, London EC1R 0AA

Lesbian and Gay Medical Association: BM GMA, London WC1N 3XX

Integrity (lesbian and gay evangelical group): PO Box 2263, London W1A 1NA

The Gay and Lesbian Humanist Association: 34 Spring Lane, Kenilworth, Warks CV8 2HB

Parents' Friend (support for parents of lesbians and gay men): c/o Voluntary Action Leeds, 34 Lupton Street, Leeds LS10 2QW Tel: 0113 267 4627

DEAF FLAG (Federation of Deaf Lesbian and Gay Groups): 7 Victoria Avenue, South Croydon, Surrey CR2 0QP

Lesbian and Gay Employment Rights (LAGER): Unit 1G, Leroy House, 436 Essex Road, London N1

Lesbian and Gay Christian Movement: Oxford House, Derbyshire Street, London E2 6HG

Lesbian and Gay Youth Movement: BM/GYM London, WC1N 3XX

REGARD (National organisation of disabled lesbians and gays): BM Regard, London WC1N 3XX

Stonewall Immigration Support Campaign: 020 7336 0620

VIGOUR (Blind and partically sighted lesbians and gays): Tel: 01701 524739 (Scotland: 01387 261679)

Positive Parenting: support for lesbian and gay foster and adoptive families: Dept. 7, 1 Newton Street, Manchester M1 1HW

appendix: Royal College of Nursing Statement

THE NURSING CARE OF LESBIANS AND GAY MEN: AN RCN STATEMENT

The Royal College of Nursing recognises through work undertaken by its members that discrimination and prejudice towards lesbian and gay patients exists in nursing.

This statement outlines the RCN's commitment to developing and promoting good nursing practice for this group of clients and to the support and assistance of any nurses who experience difficulties in developing their practice in this area.

WHAT ARE THE ACTUAL AND POTENTIAL UNMET NURSING NEEDS OF LESBIANS AND GAY MEN?

There is now a growing body of literature exploring the health care needs and experiences of lesbians and gay men. The literature demonstrates that people in this client group are exposed to many specific and additional stresses as users of the health service:

1 They have concerns that relate to homophobia or anti-lesbian and gay feelings from doctors and health care providers in general.

2 Some lesbian and gay patients fear the consequences of being open about their sexuality but also believe they cannot always get the relevant care they need if they are not open.

3 Some people fear that they may even be physically harmed if health care practitioners are homophobic and/or that a breach of confidentiality could have negative consequences for them in relation to employment, housing, child custody or future health care.

Lesbian and gay patients report experiencing negative and hostile reactions from health care practitioners when their sexual orientation is known. It has also been found that negative reactions, or even fear of such reactions, may prevent lesbians and gay men from seeking health care when it is needed.

In addition to this the literature suggests that lesbians and gay men have particular health needs which nurses should be aware of. The pressures of living as a lesbian or gay man in a society which has intense negative and condemning taboos against them may have consequences for their physical and mental health.

1 There is evidence of a much higher incidence of alcohol abuse in the lesbian and gay population which may be related to such stress.

2 There is also evidence that lesbian and gay teenagers are particularly at risk from mental and physical health problems. This is due to the lack of support they receive when trying to come to terms with their difference from accepted social norms. The high attempted suicide rate in this group is an indication of the importance which should be attached to addressing their health care needs and raising awareness amongst nurses of such needs.

3 There are suggestions that there are many other areas, as yet unresearched, in which the health status of lesbians and gay men is prejudiced; nurses need to explore these.

HOW CAN NURSES ADDRESS THESE CONCERNS?

It is clear that lesbians and gay men have specific health care needs and concerns which nurses probably do not address. A concerted response is required from the profession if we are to fulfil the collective and individual responsibilities implied by the UKCC Code of Professional Conduct in relation to this client group. As part of this response:

Nurses in clinical practice need to ensure that they never intentionally behave in a way which marginalises this client group. They must examine their behaviour towards clients to ensure that it cannot be considered as prejudicial, actively seek to raise awareness of the problem amongst colleagues and discourage unhelpful responses, and explore all possible ways of supporting and assisting lesbians and gay men using their service.

Nurses undertaking research need to develop studies of lesbians' and gay men's actual and perceived health care experiences and should establish how nurses can best meet the needs of their lesbian and gay patients.

Nurses in education need to recognise the need for the profession to be better informed and to have more positive attitudes in these areas and to design pre- and post-registration training and education strategies that recognise this.

Nurses in purchasing need to recognise the potential of the nursing contribution towards health gain for this client group and to reflect this in the contract specifications agreed with providers.

Nurses in management need to promote good practice in this area and ensure that equal opportunities in relation to service provision are adequately addressed.

Nurses also need to challenge homophobia and prejudice in the workplace wherever they encounter it.

ADVICE AND ASSISTANCE FROM THE RCN

The RCN will continue to support the development of rebust nursing practice in this area by supporting the Lesbian and Gay Nursing Needs Working Party and promoting its work. Any member who requires advice and assistance from the RCN in relation to their own practice can contact the working group via their regional office or through the Department of Nursing Policy and Practice at Headquarters (020 7409 3333).

Published by the Royal College of Nursing, the world's largest professional union of nurses.
March 1994
Order Number 000 354

Note
This statement is used by kind permission of the Royal College of Nursing and is currently under review. A fully updated version is available from the Royal College, telephone: 020 7409 3333.

references

Abbott, S. and Love, B. (1985) *Sappho was a Right-On Woman: A Liberated View of Lesbianism*. New York: Stein & Day.

Abelove, H., Barale, M. and Halperin, D. (eds) (1993) *The Lesbian and Gay Studies Reader*. London: Routledge.

Abercrombie, N., Hill, S. and Turner, B. (1988) *The Penguin Dictionary of Sociology*, 2nd edn. Harmondsworth: Penguin.

Abercrombie, N., Warde, A., Soothill, K., Urry, J. and Walby, S. (1994) *Contemporary British Society*. Cambridge: Polity.

Afshar, H. (1994) Women and the politics of fundamentalism in Islam, *Journal of Women Against Fundamentalism*, 1(5): 15–20.

Aggleton, P. (1990) *Health*. London: Routledge.

Aggleton, P., Horsley, C., Warwick, I. and Wilton, T. (1990) *AIDS: Working with Young People*. Horsham: AVERT.

Aggleton, P. and Homans, H. (1987) *Educating about AIDS*. Bristol: NHS Training Authority.

Allen, G.A. (1997) The double-edged sword of genetic determinism: Social and political agendas in genetic studies of homosexuality, 1940–1994, in V. Rosario (ed.) *Science and Homosexualities*. London: Routledge.

Alpert, H. (1988) *We Are Everywhere: Writing by and about Lesbian Parents*. Freedom, CA: The Crossing Press.

Altman, D. (1986) *AIDS and the New Puritanism*. London: Pluto Press.

Altman, D. (1993) *Homosexual Oppression and Liberation*, revised edn. New York: New York University Press.

Andersen, M. (1988) *Thinking about Women: Sociological Perspectives on Sex and Gender*. London: Macmillan.

Annandale, E. (1998) *The Sociology of Health and Medicine: A Critical Introduction*. Cambridge: Polity.

Annesley, P. (1995) Dykes and Psychs: Lesbians' Experiences and Evaluations of Clinical Psychology Services. Unpublished PsychD dissertation (Clinical Psychology), University of Sussex.

Annetts, J. and Thompson, B. (1992) Dangerous activism?, in K. Plummer (ed.) *Modern Homosexualities: Fragments of the Lesbian and Gay Experience*. London: Routledge.

Arcana, J. (1983) *Every Mother's Son: The Role of Women in the Making of Men*. London: Women's Press.

Armitage, G., Dickey, J. and Sharples, S. (1987) *Out of the Gutter: A Survey of the Treatment of Homosexuality by the Press*. London: Campaign for Press and Broadcasting Freedom.

Armstrong, D. (1989) *An Outline of Sociology as Applied to Medicine*. London: Wright.

Arnot, M. and Weiner, G. (eds) (1987) *Gender and the Politics of Schooling*. London: Hutchinson.

Ault, A. (1996) The dilemma of identity: Bi women's negotiations, in S. Seidman (ed.) *Queer Theory/Sociology*. Oxford: Blackwell.

Badden, J. (1991) Sells Papers, Ruins Lives: Homophobia and the Media, in T. Kaufmann and P. Lincoln (eds) *High Risk Lives: Lesbian and Gay Politics After THE CLAUSE*. Bridport: Prism.

Baggott, R. (1994) *Health and Health Care in Britain*. London: Macmillan.

Baldwin, S. and Twigg, J. (1991) Women and community care – reflections on a debate, in M. Maclean and D. Groves (eds) *Women's Issues in Social Policy*. London: Routledge.

Barale, M. (1991) Below the belt: (un)covering the well of loneliness, in D. Fuss (ed.) *Inside/Out: Lesbian Theories, Gay Theories*. London: Routledge.

Bard, J. and Cummins, A. (eds) (1995) *Women against Fundamentalism Education Pack*. London: WAF.

Barrett, G. (1997) Nursing and sexual health promotion: A study of nurses' perceptions of their role, practice and influencing factors. Unpublished dissertation, University of the West of England, Bristol.

Barrett, M. (1990) *Invisible Lives: The Truth about Millions of Women-Loving Women*. New York: Harper & Row.

Bassuk, E. (1985) The rest cure: Repetition or resolution of Victorian women's conflicts?, in S.R. Suleiman (ed.) *The Female Body in Western Culture: Contemporary Perspectives*. London: Harvard University Press.

Bech, H. (1992) Report from a rotten state: 'Marriage' and 'Homosexuality' in Denmark, in K. Plummer (ed.) *Modern Homosexualties: Fragments of Lesbian and Gay Experience*. London: Routledge.

Bell, D. and Valentine, G. (eds) (1995) *Mapping Desire: Geographies of Sexualities*. London: Routledge.

Berer, M. (ed.) (1998) *Reproductive Health Matters* (special issue: Sexuality), 6: 12.

Berer, M. with Ray, S. (eds) (1993) *Women and AIDS: An International Resource*. London: Pandora.

Bernard, J. (1972) *The Future of Marriage*. New York: World Publishing.

Blasius, M. and Phelan, S. (eds) (1997) *We Are Everywhere: A Historical Sourcebook of Gay and Lesbian Politics*. London: Routledge.

Boston Women's Health Book Collective (1989) *The New Our Bodies Ourselves: A Health Book by and for Women* (British edn by A. Phillips and J. Rakusen). Harmondsworth: Penguin.

Boswell, J. (1994) *The Marriage of Likeness: Same-sex Unions in Pre-Modern Europe*. London: HarperCollins.

Bowker, L. (ed.) (1998) *Masculinities and Violence*. London: Sage.

Bradstock, M. and Wakeling, L. (eds) (1987) *Words from the Same Heart*. Sydney: Hale & Iremonger.

Brandt, A. (1989) *No Magic Bullet: A Social History of Venereal Disease in the United States Since 1880*. Oxford: Oxford University Press.

Brekke, T., Davis, A. and Desai, A. (1985) *Women: a World Report*. London: Methuen.

Bremmer, J. (ed.) (1989) *From Sappho to de Sade: Moments in the History of Sexuality*. London: Routledge.

Brennan, Z. (1998) Prints put the finger on gays, *Sunday Times*, 6 February.

Braun, G. and Harris, T. (1978) *Social Origins of Depression.* London: Taristock.

Burana, L., Roxxie and Due, L. (eds) (1994) *Dagger: On Butch Women.* San Francisco: Cleis Press.

Bury, J. (1994) Women and HIV/AIDS: Medical issues, in L. Doyal, J. Naidoo and T. Wilton (eds) *AIDS: Setting a Feminist Agenda.* London: Taylor & Francis.

Butler, B. (1990) *Ceremonies of the Heart: Celebrating Lesbian Unions.* Washington: Seal Press.

Cadden, J. (1993) *Meanings of Sex Difference in the Middle Ages.* Cambridge: Cambridge University Press.

Calderone, M. and Johnson, E. (1989) *The Family Book about Sexuality.* London: Harper & Row.

Califia, P. (1994) *Public Sex: The Culture of Radical Sex.* Pittsburgh, PA: Cleis.

Califia, P. (1997) *Sex Changes: The Politics of Transgenderism.* San Francisco: Cleis.

Cameron, A., Drew, S. and Wilton, T. (1996) *Women, Weight-training and Femininity: Preliminary Report.* Bristol: University of the West of England.

Caplan, R. (ed.) (1987) *The Cultural Construction of Sexuality.* London: Routledge.

Carabine, J. (1996) Heterosexuality and social theory, in D. Richardson (ed.) *Theorising Heterosexuality: Telling it Straight.* Buckingham: Open University Press.

Carter, E. and Watney, S. (eds) (1989) *Taking Liberties: AIDS and Cultural Politics.* London: Serpent's Tail.

Cartledge, S. and Ryan, J. (eds) (1983) *Sex and Love: New Thoughts on Old Contradictions.* London: The Women's Press.

Chaplin, E. (1994) *Sociology and Visual Representation.* London: Routledge.

Chauncey, G. (1994) *Gay New York: Gender, Urban Culture and the Making of the Gay Male World, 1890–1940.* New York: Basic Books.

Clark, D. (1987) *The New Loving Someone Gay.* Berkeley, CA: Celestial Arts.

Clark, K. (1994) Is it Fundamentalism? Patterns in Islam, *Journal of Women Against Fundamentalism,* 5(1): 10–14.

Clausen, J. (1990) My interesting condition, *Outlook,* 7: 10–21.

Cockburn, C. (1985) *Machinery of Dominance: Women, Men and Technical Know-How.* London: Pluto.

Cockburn, C. (1991) *Brothers: Male Dominance and Technological Change,* 2nd edn. London: Pluto.

Colvin, M. and Hawksley, J. (1989) *Section 28: A Guide to the Law and Its Implications.* London: Liberty.

Comfort, A. (1972) *The Joy of Sex.* London: Quartet.

Comstock, G. (1991) *Violence against Lesbians and Gay Men.* New York: Columbia University Press.

Connell, R.W. (1987) *Gender and Power: Society, the Person and Sexual Politics.* Cambridge: Polity.

Connolly, L. (1996) Long-term Care and Hospice: The Special Needs of Older Gay Men and Lesbians, in K. Peterson (ed.) *Health Care for Lesbians and Gay Men: Confronting Homophobia and Heterosexism.* New York: Haworth-Press.

Cookson, S. (1988) *Housing for Lesbians and Gay Men: Report of a Conference Held 1st October 1988.* London: Housing Campaign for Single Homeless People.

Cooper, D. (1989) Positive Images in Harringey: A Struggle for Identity, in C. Jones and P. Mahony (eds) *Learning our Lines: Sexuality and Social Control in Education.* London: The Women's Press.

Coote, A. and Campbell, B. (1987) *Sweet Freedom: The Struggle for Women's Liberation.* Oxford: Blackwell.

Cossis Brown, H. (1992) Lesbians, the State and social work practice, in M. Langan and L. Day (eds) *Women, Oppression and Social Work.* London: Routledge.

Coxon, T. (1988) The numbers game – gay lifestyles, epidemiology of AIDS and social science, in P. Aggleton and H. Homans (eds) *Social Aspects of AIDS*. Lewes: Falmer Press.

Crane, P. (1982) *Gays and the Law*. London: Pluto Press.

Cruikshank, M. (1992) *The Gay and Lesbian Liberation Movement*. London: Routledge.

Darty, T. and Potter, S. (eds) (1984) *Women-Identified Women*. Pao Alto: Mayfield.

Das, R. (1996) The power of medical knowledge: Systematic misinformation and the perpetuation of lesbophobia in medical education. Paper presented at the Teaching to Promote Women's Health Conference, Women's College Hospital, University of Toronto, Canada, June.

Davidson, N. (1990) *Boys Will Be? Sex Education and Young Men*. London: Bedford Square Press.

Davies, D. and Neal, C. (eds) (1996) *Pink Therapy: A Guide for Counsellors and Therapists Working with Lesbian, Gay and Bisexual Clients*. Buckingham: Open University Press.

Davies, P., Hunt, A., Macount, M. *et al.* (1990) *Longitudinal Study of the Sexual Behaviour of Homosexual Males under the Impact of AIDS: A Final Report to the Department of Health* (Project SIGMA Working Papers). London: Department of Health.

Davies, P., Hickson, F., Weatherburn, P. and Hunt, A. (1993) *Sex, Gay Men and AIDS*. London: Falmer Press.

Deer, B. (1980) Trust is a two-way street, *New Statesman*, 27 June.

Deevey, S. (1990) Older lesbian women: An invisible minority, *Journal of Gerontological Nursing*, 16(5): 35–7.

Deitcher, D. (ed.) (1995) *Over the Rainbow: Lesbian and Gay Politics in America since Stonewall*. London: Boxtree/Channel 4.

de Lauretis, T. (1994) *The Practice of Love: Lesbian Sexuality and Perverse Desire*. Bloomington: Indiana University Press.

d'Emilio, J. and Freedman, E. (1988) *Intimate Matters: A History of Sexuality in America*. New York: Harper & Row.

Department of Education and Science (DES) (1987) *Sex Education at School* (Circular No. 11/87). London: DES.

Department of Health (DoH) (1992) *Health of the Nation*. London: The Stationery Office.

Dobson, M. (1983) At school, in B. Galloway (ed.) *Prejudice and Pride: Discrimination against Gay People in Modern Britain*. London: Routledge & Kegan Paul.

Dockery, G. (1996) *Final Report of the Research on the Sexual Health Needs of Lesbians, Bisexual Women and Women who have Sex with Women in Merseyside/Cheshire*. Liverpool: SHADY/Liverpool Health Authority.

Donoghue, E. (1993) *Passions Between Women: British Lesbian Culture 1668–1801*. London: Scarlet Press.

Douglas, C.A. (1990) *Love and Politics: Radical Feminist and Lesbian Theories*. San Francisco: ism Press.

Doyal, L. with Pennell, I. (1979) *The Political Economy of Health*. London: Pluto Press.

Doyal, L. (1995) *What Makes Women Sick: Gender and the Political Economy of Health*. London: Macmillan.

Doyal, L., Naidoo, J. and Wilton, T. (eds) (1994) *AIDS: Setting a Feminist Agenda*. London: Taylor & Francis.

Duberman, M., Vicinus, M. and Chauncey, G. (eds) (1989) *Hidden From History: Reclaiming the Gay and Lesbian Past*. London: Penguin.

Dunne, G. (1992) Difference at work: Perceptions of work from a non-heterosexual perspective, in J. Stacey, A. Pheonix and H. Hinds (eds) *Working Out: New Directions for Women's Studies*. London: Taylor & Francis.

Dunne, G.A. (1997) *Lesbian Lifestyles: Women's Work and the Politics of Sexuality.* London: Macmillan.

Dunne, G. (1998) Opting into motherhood: Lesbians blurring the boundaries and transforming the meaning of parenthood, *Working Paper No. 28.* Cambridge: Sociological Research Group, University of Cambridge.

Dunne, G. (1999) 'Lesbians do make better parents', *Stonewall Newsletter,* 8(1): 14.

Durell, A. (1983) At home, in B. Galloway (ed.) *Prejudice and Pride: Discrimination against Gay People in Modern Britain.* London: Routledge & Kegan Paul.

Dyer, R. (1989) A conversation about pornography, in S. Shepherd and M. Wallis (eds) *Coming on Strong: Gay Politics and Culture.* London: Unwin Hyman.

Eckermann, L. (1997) Foucault, embodiment and gendered subjectivities: the case of voluntary self-starvation, in A. Petersen and R. Bunton (eds) *Foucault, Health and Medicine.* London: Routledge.

Edwards, T. (1994) *Erotics and Politics: Gay Male Sexuality, Masculinity and Feminism.* London: Routledge.

Ekins, R. (1997) *Male Femaling: A Grounded Theory Approach to Cross-dressing and Sex-changing.* London: Routledge.

Ekins, R. and King, D. (eds) (1996) *Blending Genders: Social Aspects of Cross-dressing and Sex-changing.* London: Routledge.

Eliason, M.J. and Randall, C.E. (1991) Lesbian phobia in nursing students, *Western Journal of Nursing Research,* 13: 363–74.

Epstein, D. (ed.) (1994) *Challenging Lesbian and Gay Inequalities in Education.* Buckingham: Open University Press.

Epstein, J. and Straub, K. (eds) (1991) *Body Guards: The Cultural Politics of Gender Ambiguity.* London: Routledge.

Erwin, K. (1993) Interpreting the evidence: Competing paradigms and the emergence of lesbian and gay suicide as a 'social fact', *International Journal of Health Sciences,* 23(3): 437–53.

Evans, A. (1996) *We Don't Choose to be Homeless: Report of the National Inquiry into Preventing Youth Homelessness.* London: Housing Campaign for Single Homeless.

Evans, D. and Farquhar, C. (1995) *Identifying and Addressing User Views in Genito-Urinary Medicine: A Report of In-depth Research in Bristol and District.* Southampton: Institute for Health Policy Studies, Southampton University.

Ewles, L. and Simnett, I. (1985) *Promoting Health: A Practical Guide to Health Education.* Chichester: John Wiley.

Faderman, L. (1985) *Surpassing the Love of Men: Romantic Friendship and Love between Women from the Renaissance to the Present.* London: Women's Press.

Faderman, L. (1991) *Odd Girls and Twilight Lovers: A History of Lesbian Life in Twentieth-Century America.* Harmondsworth: Penguin.

Fanshaw, S. (1999) April bombings: from bullies to bombs. *Stonewall Newsletter,* 8(1), July: 2–3.

Faraday, A. (1981) Liberating lesbian research, in K. Plummer (ed.) *The Making of the Modern Homosexual.* London: Hutchinson.

Farquhar, C. (1999) Lesbian sexual health: Deconstructing research and practice. Unpublished PhD thesis, Southbank University.

Fernbach, D. (1980) Introduction, in H. Heger (ed.) *The Men with the Pink Triangle.* London: The Gay Men's Press/Bibliotek.

Fitzpatrick, R., McLean, J., Boulton, M., Hart, G. and Dawson, J. (1990) Variation in sexual behaviour in gay men, in P. Aggleton, P. Davies and G. Hart (eds) *AIDS: Individual, Cultural and Policy Dimensions.* London: Falmer Press.

Foreman, M. (ed.) (1999) *AIDS and Men: Taking Risks or Taking Responibilities?* London: Panos Institute and Zed Books.

Formani, H. (1991) *Men. The Darker Continent*. London: Mandarin.

Foucault, M. (1976) *The History of Sexuality: An Introduction*. Harmondsworth: Penguin.

Fox, N. (1993) *Postmodernism, Sociology and Health*. Buckingham: Open University Press.

Fraser, N. (1989) *Unruly Practices: Power, Discourse and Gender in Contemporary Theory*. Cambridge: Polity Press.

French, M. (1992) *The War Against Women*. London: Hamish Hamilton.

Fuss, D. (1989) *Essentially Speaking: Feminism, Nature and Difference*. London: Routledge.

Gabe, J., Kelleher, D. and Williams, G. (eds) (1994) *Challenging Medicine*. London: Routledge.

Galloway, B. (ed.) (1983) *Prejudice and Pride: Discrimination against Gay People in Modern Britain*. London: Routledge & Kegan Paul.

Gardiner, B. (2000) Slight of Hand, *The Guardian* (*G2* supplement), 31 March.

Gartrell, N., Hamilton, J., Banks, A. *et al.* (1996) The national lesbian family study: Interviews with prospective mothers, *American Journal of Orthopsychiatry*, 66(2): 272–81.

Gastaldo, D. (1997) Is health education good for you? Rethinking health education through the concept of bio-power, in A. Petersen and R. Bunton (eds) *Foucault, Health and Medicine*. London: Routledge.

Gavey, N. (1992) Technologies and effects of heterosexual coercion, in C. Kitzinger, S. Wilkinson and R. Perkins (eds) *Feminism and Psychology*, 2(3) (special issue: Heterosexuality): 325–52.

George, V. and Miller, S. (eds) (1994) *Social Policy Towards 2000: Squaring the Welfare Circle*. London: Routledge.

Gergen, K.J. (1985) The social constructionist movement in modern psychology, *American Psychologist*, 40: 266–75.

Gibson, M. (1997) Clitoral corruption: Body metaphors and American doctors' construction of female homosexuality, in V. Rosario (ed.) *Science and Homosexualities*. London: Routledge.

Giddens, A. (1992) *The Transformation of Intimacy: Sexuality, Love and Eroticism in Modern Societies*. Cambridge: Polity.

Giddens, A. (1997) *Sociology*, 3rd edn. Cambridge: Polity.

Gilman, S. (1995) *Health and Illness: Images of Difference*. London: Reaktion.

Gomez, J. and Smith, B. (1990) Taking the home out of homophobia: Black lesbian health, in E.C. White (ed.) *The Black Women's Health Handbook: Speaking for Ourselves*. Washington: Sea.

Gomez, J., Peck, D., Segrest, M. and Deitcher, D. (eds) (1995) *Over the Rainbow: Lesbian and Gay Politics in America since Stonewall*. London: Channel 4/Boxtree.

Gonsiorek, J. (1988) Current and future developments in gay/lesbian affirmative mental health practice, in M. Shernoff and W. Scott (eds) *The Sourcebook on Gay/ Lesbian Healthcare*. Washington: National Lesbian and Gay Healthcare Foundation.

Gonsiorek, J. and Weinrich, J. (eds) (1991) *Homosexuality: Research Implications for Public Policy*. London: Sage.

Gough, J. (1989) Theories of sexual identity and the masculinization of the gay man, in S. Shepherd and M. Wallis (eds) *Coming on Strong: Gay Politics and Culture*. London: Unwin Hyman.

Graham, H. (1993) *Hardship and Health in Women's Lives*. London: Harvester Wheatsheaf.

Graham, H. (1997) Finding a home, in C. Ungerson and M. Kember (eds) *Women and Social Policy: A Reader*. London: Macmillan.

Grahn, J. (1984) *Another Mother Tongue: Gay Words, Gay Worlds*. Boston: Beacon Press.

Grau, G. (1995) *Hidden Holocaust? Gay and Lesbian Persecution in Germany 1933–45.* London: Cassell.

Greater London Council (GLC) (1985) *Changing the World – a London Charter for Gay and Lesbian Rights.* London: GLC.

Green, T., Harrison, B. and Innes, J. (1996) *Not for Turning: An Enquiry into the Ex-Gay Movement.* Camberley: published jointly by the authors.

Greenberg, D. (1988) *The Construction of Homosexuality.* Chicago: University of Chicago Press.

Greer, G. (1970) *The Female Eunuch.* London: Paladin.

Griffin, G., Stein, N. and de Pinho, H. (1998) *Divided in Ourselves: Cape Town Gay Men, Lesbians and Bisexuals Talk about their Health Education and Care Needs.* Cape Town: Triangle Project.

Griffin, K. and Mulholland, L. (eds) (1997) *Lesbian Motherhood in Europe.* London: Cassell.

Griggs, C. (1998) *S/He: Changing Sex and Changing Clothes.* Oxford: Berg.

Gullette, M. (1997) Menopause as magic marker: Discursive consolidation in the United States and strategies for cultural combat, in P. Komesaroff, P. Rothfield and J. Daly (eds) *Reinterpreting Menopause: Cultural and Philosophical Issues.* London: Routledge.

Haeberle, E.J. (1989) Swastika, pink triangle and yellow star: The destruction of sexology and the persecution of homosexuals in Nazi Germany, in M.B. Duberman, M. Vicinus and G. Chauncey Jnr (eds) *Hidden from History: Reclaiming the Gay and Lesbian Past.* Harmondsworth: Penguin.

Halberstam, J. (1998) *Female Masculinities.* London: Duke University Press.

Halberstam, J. and Volcano, D.L. (1999) *The Drag King Book.* London: Serpent's Tail.

Haldeman, D. (1991) Sexual orientation conversion therapy for gay men and lesbians: A scientific examination, in J. Gonsiorek and J. Weinrich (eds) *Homosexuality: Research Implications for Public Policy.* London: Sage.

Hale, S. ([1868] 1972) *Manners: Or, Happy Homes and Good Society all the Year Round.* New York: Arno Press.

Hall, J. (1993) An exploration of lesbians' images of recovery from alcohol problems, in P. Noerager Stern (ed.) *Lesbian Health: What are the Issues?* London: Taylor & Francis.

Hall, R. (1927) *The Well of Loneliness.* London: Pandora.

Hall Carpenter Archives (Lesbian Oral History Group) (1989) *Inventing Ourselves: Lesbian Life Stories.* London: Routledge.

Halperin, D. (1989) Sex before sexuality: Pederasty, politics and power in classical Athens, in M.B. Duberman, M. Vicinus and G. Chauncey Jnr (eds) *Hidden from History: Reclaiming the Gay and Lesbian Past.* Harmondsworth: Penguin.

Ham, C. (1992) *Health Policy in Britain: The Politics and Organisation of the National Health Service.* London: Macmillan.

Hamer, D. and Copeland, P. (1994) *The Science of Desire: The Search for the Gay Gene and the Biology of Behavior.* New York: Simon & Schuster.

Hansen, S. and Jensen, J. (1971) *The Little Red School Book.* London: Stage 1.

Harding, J. (1997) Bodies at risk: Sex, surveillance and hormone replacement therapy, in A. Petersen and R. Bunton (eds) *Foucault, Health and Medicine.* London: Routledge.

Hardman, K. (1996) Social workers' attitudes to lesbian clients. Unpublished dissertation, University of London.

Hardman, K. (1997) Social workers' attitudes to lesbian clients, *British Journal of Social Work,* 27: 545–63.

Hargaden, H. and Llewellin, S. (1996) Lesbian and gay parenting issues, in D. Davies and C. Neal (eds) *Pink Therapy: A Guide for Counsellors and Therapists Working with Lesbian, Gay and Bisexual Clients*. Buckingham: Open University Press.

Hart, N. (1985) *The Sociology of Health and Medicine*. Ormskirk: Causeway.

Hartouni, V. (1997) *Cultural Conceptions: On Reproductive Technologies and the Remaking of Life*. Minneapolis: University of Minnesota Press.

Harvard Law Review (eds) (1989) *Sexual Orientation and the Law*. Cambridge, MA: Harvard University Press.

Harwood, L. (1998) In the pink? Lesbian students' experiences of social work education, *Social Work Education*, 17(2): 157–71.

Hasbany, R. (ed.) (1989) *Homosexuality and Religion*. New York: Harrington Park Press.

Heger, H. (ed.) (1980) *The Men with the Pink Triangle*. London: The Gay Men's Press/Bibliotek.

Heise, L. (1997) Violence, sexuality and women's lives, in R. Lancaster and M. de Leonardo (eds) *The Gender Sexuality Reader: Culture, History, Political Economy*. London: Routledge.

Helminiak, D. (1994) *What the Bible Really Says about Homosexuality*. San Francisco, CA: Alamo Square Press.

Hemmings, S. (1986) Overdose of doctors, in S. O'Sullivan (ed.) *Women's Health: A Spare Rib Reader*. London: Pandora.

Hepburn, C. and Guttierrez, B. (1988) *Alive and Well: A Lesbian Health Guide*. Freedom, CA: The Crossing Press.

Herdt, G. (1989) *Gay and Lesbian Youth*. New York: Haworth Press.

Hevey, D. (1992) *The Creatures that Time Forgot: Photography and Disability Imagery*. London: Routledge.

Hidalgo, H. (ed.) (1995) *Lesbians of Colour: Social and Human Services*. New York: Haworth Press.

Hidalgo, H., Petersen, T. and Woodman, J. (eds) (1985) *Lesbian and Gay Issues: A Resource Manual for Social Workers*. Washington, DC: National Association of Social Workers.

Hoagland, S.L. (1988) *Lesbian Ethics: Towards New Values*. Palo Alto, CA: Institute of Lesbian Studies.

Hobson, B.M. (1987) *Uneasy Virtue: The Politics of Prostitution and the American Reform Tradition*. New York: Basic Books.

Holmes, S. (ed.) (1988) *Testimonies: A Collection of Lesbian Coming Out Stories*. Boston, MA: Allyson.

Hoolaghan, T., Blache, G. and Pidock, J. (1993) *The Role of General Practitioners in HIV Prevention: Findings from a Questionnaire Survey*. London: The Health Promotion in General Practice Project, Camden and Islington Health Promotion Service.

Hubback, J. (1957) *Wives Who Went to College*. London: Heinemann.

Humphreys, L. (1970) *The Tearoom Trade*. London: Duckworth.

Hunt, A. and Davies, P. (1991) What is a sexual encounter?, in P. Aggleton, G. Hart and P. Davies (eds) *AIDS: Responses, Interventions and Care*. Brighton: Falmer Press.

Ilett, R. (1995) Lesbian health at the fore, *Gay Scotland*, 92 (May): 7.

Institute of Medicine (National Academy of Sciences) (1986) *Mobilizing Against Aids: The Unfinished Story of a Virus*. Cambridge, MA: Harvard University Press.

Institute of Medicine (1999) *Lesbian Health: Current Assessment and Directions for the Future*. Washington, DC: National Academy Press.

International Lesbian and Gay Association (eds) (1988) *The Second ILGA Pink Book: A Global View of Lesbian and Gay Liberation and Oppression*. Utrecht: University of Utrecht.

Isay, R. (1989) *Being Homosexual: Gay Men and Their Development*. Harmondsworth: Penguin.

Isherwood, L. and Stuart, E. (1998) *Introducing Body Theology*. Sheffield: Sheffield Academic Press.

Jackson, C. (1998) Diagnosis homophobic: The experiences of lesbians, gay men and bisexuals in mental health services, *Women and Mental Health Forum*, 4, May: 3–5.

James, T., Harding, I. and Corbett, K. (1994) Biased care? Lesbians and gay men, *Nursing Times*, 90(51) (December): 28–31.

Jay, K. (ed.) (1995) *Dyke Life From Growing Up to Growing Old: A Celebration of the Lesbian Experience*. London: Pandora.

Jeffreys, S. (1990) *Anticlimax: A Feminist Perspective on the Sexual Revolution*. London: The Women's Press.

Jennings White, H. (1925) *Psychological Causes of Homoerotism and Inversion*. London: British Society for the Study of Sex Psychology.

Jessop, J. and Thorogood, N. (1989) Sexuality and health, *Radical Community Medicine*, Winter: 11–17.

Johnston, J. (1973) *Lesbian Nation*. New York: Touchstone.

Jones, H. (1994) *Health and Society in Twentieth-Century Britain*. London: Longman.

Jones, L. (1994) *The Social Context of Health and Health Work*. London: Macmillan.

Katz, J.N. (1983) *Gay/Lesbian Almanac: A New Documentary*. New York: Harper & Row.

Kaufmann, T. and Lincoln, P. (eds) (1991) *High Risk Lives: Lesbian and Gay Politics After THE CLAUSE*. Bridport: Prism.

Kayal, P. (1993) *Bearing Witness: Gay Men's Health Crisis and the Politics of AIDS*. Boulder, CO: Westview Press.

Kember, M. (1997) Lone mothers: Introduction, in C. Ungerson and M. Kember (eds) *Women and Social Policy: A Reader*. London: Macmillan.

Kenen, S. (1997) Who counts when you're counting homosexuals? Hormones and homosexuality in mid-twentieth-century America, in V. Rosario (ed.) *Science and Homosexualities*. London: Routledge.

Kenney, J. and Tash, D. (1993) Lesbian childbearing couples' dilemmas and decisions, in P. Noergaer Stern (ed.) *Lesbian Health: What are the Issues?* London: Taylor & Francis.

Kidd, M. (1999) The bearded lesbian, in J. Arthurs and J. Grimshaw (eds) *Women's Bodies: Discipline and Transgression*. London: Cassell.

King, A., Beazley, R., Warren, W. *et al.* (1989) *Canada Youth and AIDS Study*. Kingston: Queens' University at Kingston.

King, E. (1993) *Safety in Numbers: Safer Sex and Gay Men*. London: Cassell.

Kinsey, A.C., Pomeroy, W.B. and Martin, C.E. (1948) *Sexual Behaviour in the Human Male*. Philadelphia: W.B. Sanders.

Kirkpatrick, A. and Kirkpatrick, D. (1987) *AIDS*. Edinburgh: Chambers.

Kitzinger, C. (1987) *The Social Construction of Lesbianism*. London: Sage.

Kramer, J.L. (1995) Bachelor farmers and spinsters: Gay and lesbian identities and communities in rural North Dakota, in D. Bell and G. Valentine (eds) *Mapping Desire: Geographies of Sexualities*. London: Routledge.

Kramer, L. (1990) *Reports from the Holocaust: The Making of an AIDS Activist*. Harmondsworth: Penguin.

Lancaster, R. (1995) 'That we should all turn queer?' Homosexual stigma in the making of manhood and the breaking of a revolution in Nicaragua, in R. Parker and J. Gagnon (eds) *Conceiving Sexuality: Approaches to Sex Research in a Postmodern World*. London: Routledge.

Lancaster, R. and di Leonardo, M. (eds) (1997) *The Gender Sexuality Reader: Culture, History, Political Economy*. London: Routledge.

Langan, M. (1997) Who cares? Women in the mixed economy of care, in C. Ungerson and M. Kember (eds) *Women and Social Policy: A Reader*. London: Macmillan.

Lee, N'T., Murphy, D. and Ucelli, J. (1995) Whose kids? Our kids!, *Journal of Women Against Fundamentalism*, 6(1): 26–32.

Lesbian History Group (1989) *Not a Passing Phase: Reclaiming Lesbians in History 1840–1985*. London: The Women's Press.

LeVay, S. (1993) *The Sexual Brain*. Cambridge, MA: Massachusetts Institute of Technology Press.

LeVay, S. (1996) *Queer Science: The Uses and Abuses of Research into Homosexuality*. Cambridge, MA: Massachusetts Institute of Technology Press.

Levine, M. and Leonard, R. (1985) Discrimination against lesbians in the work force, in E. Freedman, B. Gelpi, S. Johnson and K. Weston (eds) *The Lesbian Issue: Essays from SIGNS*. Chicago: University of Chicago Press.

Leznoff, M. and Westley, W.A. (1967) The homosexual community, in J. Gagnon and W. Simon (eds) *Sexual Deviance*. New York: Harper & Row.

Llewellyn-Jones, D. (1985) *Herpes, AIDS and Other Sexually Transmitted Diseases*. London: Faber & Faber.

Lobell, K. (1986) *Naming the Violence: Speaking out about Lesbian Battering*. Seattle: Seal Press.

London Gay Teenage Group (LGTG) (1984) *Something to Tell You: The Experiences and Needs of Young Lesbians and Gay Men in London*. London: LGTG.

Lucia-Hoagland, S. and Penelope, J. (eds) (1988) *For Lesbians Only: A Separatist Anthology*. London: Onlywomen Press.

Lupton, D. (1996) *The Imperative of Health: Public Health and the Regulated Body*. London: Sage.

Lynch, L. and Woods, A. (eds) (1996) *Off the Rag: Lesbians Writing on Menopause*. Norwich, VT: New Victoria Publishers.

Lyon-Martin Women's Health Services (1993) *Lesbian Health Care: Information, Research and Reports*. San Francisco, CA: Lyon-Martin Women's Health Services.

Macdonald, B. with Rich, C. (1985) *Look Me in the Eye: Old Women, Age and Ageism*. London: The Women's Press.

MacInnes, J. (1998) *The End of Masculinity*. Buckingham: Open University Press.

Macionis, J. and Plummer, K. (1997) *Sociology: A Global Introduction*. London: Prentice Hall Europe.

Maclean, M. and Groves, D. (eds) (1991) *Women's Issues in Social Policy*. London: Routledge.

Malos, E. (1980) The Politics of Housework. London: Allison & Busby.

Marshall, J. (1983) The medical profession, in B. Galloway (ed.) *Prejudice and Pride: Discrimination against Gay People in Modern Britain*. London: Routledge & Kegan Paul.

Martin, E. (1987) *The Woman in The Body: A Cultural Analysis of Reproduction*. Milton Keynes: Open University Press.

Mason, A. and Palmer, A. (1996) *Queer Bashing: A National Survey of Hate Crimes Against Lesbians and Gay Men*. London: Stonewall.

McClintock, A. (1995) *Imperial Leather: Race, Gender and Sexuality in the Colonial Contest*. London: Routledge.

McClure, R. and Vespry, A. (eds) (1994) *Lesbian Health Guide*. Toronto: Queer Press.

McCormick, I. (ed.) (1997) *Secret Sexualities: A Sourcebook of 17th and 18th Century Writings*. London: Routledge.

McFarlane, L. (1998) *Diagnosis Homophobic: The Experiences of Lesbians, Gay Men and Bisexuals in Mental Health Services*. London: PACE.

McIntosh, M. (1968) The Homosexual Role. Reprinted in K. Plummer (ed.) (1981) *The Making of the Modern Homosexual*. London: Hutchinson.

Menasche, A. (1999) *Leaving the Life: Lesbians, Ex-Lesbians and the Heterosexual Imperative*. London: Onlywomen Press.

Merck, M. (1993) *PerVersions: Deviant Readings*. London: Virago.

Mernissi, F. (1986) Femininity as subversion: Reflections on the Muslim concept of Nushuz, in D. Eck and D. Jain (eds) *Speaking of Faith: Cross-Cultural Perspectives on Women, Religion and Social Change*. London: The Women's Press.

Miedzian, M. (1992) *Boys Will Be Boys: Breaking the Link Between Masculinity and Violence*. London: Virago.

Millar, J. (1997) State, family and personal responsibility: The changing balance for lone mothers in the UK, in C. Ungerson and M. Kember (eds) *Women and Social Policy: A Reader*. London: Macmillan.

Miller, N. (1995) *Out of the Past: Gay and Lesbian History from 1869 to the Present*. London: Vintage.

Moon, G. and Gillespie, R. (eds) (1995) *Society and Health: An Introduction to Social Science for Health Professionals*. London: Routledge.

Moore, T. (1945) The pathogenesis and treatment of homosexual disorders: a digest of some pertinent evidence, *Journal of Personality*, 14 (Sept): 56–7.

Morgan, R. (ed.) (1984) *Sisterhood is Global*. Harmondsworth: Penguin.

Mort, F. ([1987] 1999) *Dangerous Sexualities: Medico-moral Politics in England Since 1830*. London: Routledge & Kegan Paul.

Mugglestone, J. (1999) *Report of the Bolton and Wigan Lesbian Health Needs Assessment: 'Are You Sure You Don't Need Contraception?'* Bolton: Bolton Specialist Health Promotion Service.

Muir-Mackenzie, A. and Orme, K. (eds) (1996) *Health of the Lesbian, Gay and Bisexual Nation: 1996 Conference Offical Report*. Plymouth: The Harbour Centre.

Murray, T. and McClure, M. (1995) Gay and lesbian Christian apologetics, *Journal of Women Against Fundamentalism*, 7(1): 40–2.

Naidoo, J. and Wills, J. (1994) *Health Promotion: Foundations for Practice*. London: Balliere Tyndall.

National AIDS Trust (NAT) (1991) *Living For Tomorrow* (Report of the NAT Youth Initiative). London: NAT.

National Lesbian and Gay Survey (1992) *What a Lesbian Looks Like: Writings by Lesbians on their Lives and Lifestyles*. London: Routledge.

Neild, S. and Pearson, R. (eds) (1992) *Women Like Us*. London: The Women's Press.

Nettleton, S. (1995) *The Sociology of Health and Illness*. Cambridge: Polity.

Neville, R. (1971) *Playpower*. London: Paladin.

Nelkin, D. and Lindee, S. (1995) The Media-ted gene: Stories of gender and race, in J. Terry and J. Urla (eds) *Deviant Bodies: Critical Perspectives on Difference in Science and Popular Culture*. Bloomington, IN: Indiana University Press.

Nestle, J. (1987) *A Restricted Country: Essays and Short Stories*. London: Pandora.

Nicholas, J. and Howard, J. (1998) Better to be dead than gay? Depression, suicidal ideation and attempts among a sample of gay and straight-identified males aged 18–24. Paper presented at Out of the Blues: Depression in Young People, the Agenda for the Future, Macquarie University, Sydney, 6–9 November.

Nichols, M. (1988) Lesbian relationships and lesbian sexuality: Implications for the study of sexuality and gender, in M. Shernoff and W. Scott (eds) *The Sourcebook on Lesbian/Gay Health Care*. Washington: National Lesbian and Gay Health Foundation.

Nugent, R. and Gramick, J. (1998) Homosexuality: Protestant, Catholic and Jewish Issues, A Fishbone Tale, in R. Hasbany (ed.) *Homosexuality and Religion*. New York: Harrington Park Press.

Oakley, A. (1972) *Sex, Gender and Society*. London: Temple Smith.

O'Rourke, R. (1989) *Reflecting on* The Well of Loneliness. London: Routledge.

Palmer, A. (1996) Britain, in R. Rosenblum (ed.) *Unspoken Rules: Sexual Orientation and Women's Human Rights*. London: International Gay and Lesbian Human Rights Commission/Cassell.

Panos Institute (1990) *Triple Jeopardy: Women and AIDS*. London: Panos Publications.

Pateman, C. (1992) Equality, difference, subordination: the politics of motherhood and women's citizenship, in G. Bock and S. James (eds) *Beyond Equality and Difference: Citizenship, Feminist Politics and Female Subjectivity*. London: Routledge.

Patton, C. (1985) *Sex and Germs: The Politics of AIDS*. Boston: South End Press.

Patton, C. (1994) *Last Served? Gendering the HIV Pandemic*. London: Taylor & Francis.

Payne, S. (1991) *Women, Health and Poverty: An Introduction*. London: Harvester Wheatsheaf.

Pennell Initiative (1998) *The Pennell Report On Women's Health: Positive Steps for Later Life*. London: Pennell Initiative (University of Manchester).

Petersen, A. and Bunton, R. (eds) (1997) *Foucault, Health and Medicine*. London: Routledge.

Petersen, K. (ed.) (1996) *Health Care for Lesbians and Gay Men*. New York: Haworth.

Pharr, S. (1988) *Homophobia: a Weapon of Sexism*. Little Rock: Chardon Press.

Pieterse, J.N. (1994) Fundamentalism discourses: enemy images, *Women Against Fundamentalism Journal*, 1(5): 2–6.

Pillard, R. (1997) The search for a genetic influence on sexual orientation, in V. Rosario (ed.) *Science and Homosexualities*. London: Routledge.

Plummer, K. (1981) Building a sociology of homosexuality, in K. Plummer (ed.) *The Making of the Modern Homosexual*. London: Hutchinson.

Plummer, K. (ed.) (1992) *Modern Homosexualities: Fragments of Lesbian and Gay Experience*. London: Routledge.

Plummer, K. (1995) *Telling Sexual Stories: Power, Change and Social Worlds*. London: Routledge.

Pollinger Haas, A. (1994) Lesbian health issues: An overview, in A. Dan (ed.) *Reframing Women's Health*. Thousand Oaks, CA: Sage.

Porter, K. and Weeks, J. (eds) (1991) *Between the Acts: Lives of Homosexual Men 1885–1967*. London: Routledge.

Porter, R. (1997) *The Greatest Benefit to Mankind: A Medical History of Humanity from Antiquity to the Present*. London: HarperCollins.

Powell, V. (1998) Christian onslaught on gay rights, *Gay Times*, May: 43.

Proctor, R. (1995) The destruction of 'lives not worth living', in J. Terry and J. Urla (eds) *Deviant Bodies: Critical Perspectives on Difference in Science and Popular Culture*. Indianapolis, IN: Indiana University Press.

Rafkin, L. (ed.) (1990) *Different Mothers: Sons and Daughters of Lesbians Talk about their Lives*. San Francisco, CA: Cleis Press.

Ramet, S.P. (ed.) (1996) *Gender Reversals and Gender Cultures*. London: Routledge.

Ranade, W. (1994) *A Future for the NHS? Health Care in the 1990s*. London: Longman.

Rayner, P.H.W. (1994) Medical concern prompts lifestyle judgements (letter), *British Medical Journal*, 308: 854.

Reid, R. (1995) 'Death of the family', or, keeping human beings human, in J. Halberstam and I. Livingstone (eds) *Posthuman Bodies*. Indianapolis, IN: Indiana University Press.

Reinfelder, M. (ed.) (1995) *Amazon to Zami: Towards a Global Lesbian Feminism*. London: Cassell.

Remafidi, G., Farrow, J.A. and Deisher, R.W. (1991) Risk factors for attempted suicide in gay and bisexual youth, *Paediatrics*, 87(6): 869–75.

Renzetti, C. (1992) *Violent Betrayal: Partner Abuse in Lesbian Relationships*. London: Sage.

Reuben, D. (1969) *Everything You Always Wanted to Know about Sex*. New York: Bantam.

Reynaud, E. (1981) *Holy Virility: The Social Construction of Masculinity*. London: Pluto.

Richardson, D. (1989) *Women and the AIDS Crisis*. London: Pandora.

Richardson, D. (1993) *Women, Motherhood and Childrearing*. London: Macmillan.

Richardson, D. (1994) Inclusions and exclusions: Lesbians, HIV and AIDS, in L. Doyal, J. Naidoo and T. Wilton (eds) *AIDS: Setting a Feminist Agenda*. London: Taylor & Francis.

Richardson, D. (ed.) (1996) *Theorising Heterosexuality: Telling it Straight*. Buckingham: Open University Press.

Richardson, D. (1998) Sexuality and citizenship, *Sociology*, 32(1): 83–100.

Robertson, M. (1993) Lesbians as an invisible minority in the health services arena, in P. Stern (ed.) *Lesbian Health: What are the Issues?* London: Taylor & Francis.

Rochlin, M. (1992) Heterosexual questionnaire, in W.J. Blumenfeld (ed.) *Homophobia: How We All Pay the Price*. Boston, MA: Beacon Press.

Rosario, V. (ed.) (1997) *Science and Homosexualities*. London: Routledge.

Rose, P. (1993) Out in the open? How do nurses treat their patients and colleagues who are lesbians?, *Nursing Times*, 89(30): 50–2.

Rosenblum, R. (1996) *Unspoken Rules: Sexual Orientation and Women's Human Rights*. London: Cassell.

Royal College of Nursing (RCN) (1994) *The Nursing Care of Lesbians and Gay Men: An RCN Statement*. London: RCN.

Royal College of Nursing (RCN) (1998) *Guidance for Nurses on 'Next-of-kin' for Lesbian and Gay Patients and Children with Lesbian or Gay Parents*, Issues in nursing and health no. 47. London: RCN.

Rule, J. (1985) *A Hot-Eyed Moderate*. Tallahassee, FL: Naiad.

Ruse, M. (1988) *Homosexuality: A Philosophical Inquiry*. Oxford: Basil Blackwell.

Saffron, L. (1994) *Challenging Conceptions: Planning a Family by Self-insemination*. London: Cassell.

Saffron, L. (1996) *What about the Children? Sons and Daughters of Lesbian and Gay Parents Talk about their Lives*. London: Cassell.

Sahgal, G. and Yuval-Davis, N. (eds) (1992) *Refusing Holy Orders: Women and Fundamentalism in Britain*. London: Virago.

SAMOIS (eds) (1981) *Coming to Power: Writings and Graphics on Lesbian S.M.* Boston, MA: Alyson Press.

Sanders, S. and Spraggs, G. (1989) Section 28 and education, in C. Jones and P. Mahoney (eds) *Learning Our Lines: Sexuality and Social Control in Education*. London: The Women's Press.

Sanderson, T. (1995) *Mediawatch: The Treatment of Male and Female Homosexuality in the British Media*. London: Cassell.

Saraga, E. (ed.) (1998) *Embodying the Social: Constructions of Difference*. London: Routledge/The Open University.

Sarup, M. (1993) *An Introductory Guide to Post-Structuralism and Postmodernism*. London: Harvester Wheatsheaf.

Savage, J. (1987) *Nurses, Gender and Sexuality*. London: Heinemann.

Sawday, J. (1995) *The Body Emblazoned: Dissection and the Human Body in Renaissance Culture*. London: Routledge.

Sayce, L. and Perkins, R. (1998) Some thoughts on recent alarm about 'paedophiles', *Women and Mental Health Forum*, 4, May: 16.

Schulman, S. (1994) *My American Life: Lesbian and Gay Life During the Reagan/Bush Years*. London: Cassell.

Schwanberg, S.L. (1990) Attitudes to homosexuality in American health care literature 1983–1987, *Journal of Homosexuality*, 19(3): 117–37.

Schwartz, P. and Rutter, V. (1998) *The Gender of Sexuality*. London: Pine Forge Press.

Schwartz, R.L. (1993) New alliances, strange bedfellows: Lesbians, gay men and AIDS, in A. Stein (ed.) *Sisters, Sexperts, Queers: Beyond the Lesbian Nation*. Harmondsworth: Penguin.

Scruton, R. (1986) *Sexual Desire*. London: Weidenfeld & Nicolson.

Sears, J. (1991) *Growing up Gay in the South: Race, Gender and Journeys of the Spirit*. New York: Haworth Press.

Segal, L. (1994) *Straight Sex: The Politics of Pleasure*. London: Virago.

Segrest, M. (1995) Visibility and backlash, in D. Deitcher (ed.) *Over the Rainbow: Lesbian and Gay Politics in America since Stonewall*. London: Boxtree/Channel 4.

Seidman, S. (ed.) (1996) *Queer Theory/Sociology*. Oxford: Blackwell.

Shakespeare, T., Gillespie-Sells, K. and Davies, D. (eds) (1996) *The Sexual Politics of Disability: Untold Desires*. London: Cassell.

Sheffield Health (1996) *Lesbian Health Needs Assessment: Report of a Participatory Research Study*. Sheffield: Healthy Sheffield Team.

Shepherd, S. (1989) Gay sex spy orgy: The state's need for queers, in S. Shepherd and M. Wallis (eds) *Coming on Strong: Gay Politics and Culture*. London: Unwin & Hyman.

Shernoff, M. (1988) Sexual exclusivity, nonexclusivity and emotional bonding in male couples, in M. Shernoff and W. Scott (eds) *The Sourcebook on Lesbian/Gay Health Care*. Washington, DC: National Lesbian and Gay Health Foundation.

Shernoff, M. and Scott, W. (eds) (1988) *The Sourcebook on Lesbian/Gay Health Care*. Washington, DC: National Lesbian and Gay Health Foundation.

Shilts, R. (1987) *And the Band Played On: Politics, People and the AIDS Epidemic*. New York: St Martin's Press.

Shiers (1988) One step to heaven? in B. Cant and S. Hemmings (eds) *Radical Records: Thirty Years of Lesbian and Gay History*. London: Routledge.

Short, R. (1997) The road to reproductive health, *Medical Research Council News*, 75: 1.

Showalter, E. (1987) *The Female Malady: Women, Madness and English Culture, 1830–1980*. London: Virago.

Signorile, M. (1993) *Queer in America: Sex, the Media and the Closets of Power*. New York: Abacus.

Silverstein, C. (1991) Psychological and medical treatments of homosexuality, in J. Gonsiorek and J. Weinrich (eds) *Homosexuality: Research Implications for Public Policy*. London: Sage.

Simpson, M. (1994) *Male Impersonators: Men Performing Masculinity*. London: Cassell.

Singer, B. and Deschamps, D. (eds) (1994) *Gay and Lesbian Stats: A Pocket Guide of Facts and Figures*. New York: The New Press.

Smart, C. and Smart, B. (eds) (1978) *Women, Sexuality and Social Control*. London: Routledge and Kegan Paul.

Smith, A.M. (1992) Resisting the erasure of lesbian sexuality: A challenge for queer activism', in K. Plummer (ed.) *Modern Homosexualities: Fragments of the Lesbian and Gay Experience*. London: Routledge.

Smith, A.M. (1994) *New Right Discourse on Race and Sexuality: Britain, 1968–1990*. Cambridge: Cambridge University Press.

Smith, F.B. (1979) *The People's Health*. New York: Holmes & Meier.

Smyth, C. (1992) *Lesbians Talk Queer Notions*. London: Scarlet Press.

Somerset Health Authority (1998) *Sexual Health Strategy*. Taunton: Somerset Health Authority.

Stacey, J. (1997) The neo-family-values campaign, in R. Lancaster and M. de Leonardo (eds) *The Gender Sexuality Reader: Culture, History, Political Economy*. London: Routledge.

Steel, M. (1998) Out in the cold, *Diva*, May: 32–5.

Stein, E. (ed.) (1990) *Forms of Desire: Sexual Orientation and the Social Constructionist Controversy*. London: Routledge.

Stern, P.N. (ed.) (1993) *Lesbian Health: What are the Issues?* London: Taylor & Francis.

Stevens, P. (1993) Lesbian health care research: A review of the literature from 1970 to 1990, in P.N. Stern (ed.) *Lesbian Health, What Are the Issues?* London: Taylor & Francis.

Stewart, F. (1996) Mounting a challenge: Young women, heterosexuality and safe sex. Unpublished PhD thesis, La Trobe University, Australia.

Stewart, M. (1997) We just want to be ordinary: Lesbian parents talk about their birth experiences. Unpublished Master's dissertation, University of the West of England, Bristol.

Stewart, W. (1995) *Cassell's Queer Companion*. London: Cassell.

Stoltenberg, J. (1989) *Refusing to Be a Man*. London: Fontana.

Stoneham Housing Association (1996) *Hearing Young People*. London: National Housing Federation.

Stonewall (1999) *Stonewall Newsletter*, 8(1), July: 2–3.

Strong, B., DeVault, C. and Sayad, B.V. (1996) *Core Concepts in Human Sexuality*. London: Mayfield.

Stuart, E. (1992) *Daring to Speak Love's Name: A Gay and Lesbian Prayer Book*. London: Hamish Hamilton.

Sutcliffe, P. (1999) Rock Out, *Q*, February: 76–83.

Symonds, J. (1984) *Sexual Inversion*. New York: Bell (first published 1928).

Symonds, A. and Hunt, S. (1996) *The Midinge and Society: Perspectives, Policies and Practices*. London.

Tannahill, R. (1992) *Sex in History*. New York: Scarborough House.

Tatchell, P. (1990) *Out in Europe: A Guide to Lesbian and Gay Rights in 30 European Countries*. London: Rouge/Channel 4.

Tatchell, P. (1992) Equal rights for all: Strategies for lesbian and gay equality in Britain, in K. Plummer (ed.) *Modern Homosexualities: Fragments of Lesbian and Gay Experience*. London: Routledge.

Terry, J. (1995) Anxious slippages between 'us' and 'them': A brief history of the scientific search for homosexual bodies, in J. Terry and J. Urla (eds) *Deviant Bodies: Critical Perspectives on Difference in Science and Popular Culture*. Bloomington: Indiana University Press.

Terry, J. (1997) The seductive power of science in the making of deviant subjectivities, in V. Rosario (ed.) *Science and Homosexualities*. New York: Routledge.

Terry, J. and Urla, J. (eds) (1995) *Deviant Bodies: Critical Perspectives on Difference in Science and Popular Culture*. Bloomington: Indiana University Press.

Thompson, M. (1987) *Gay Spirit: Myth and Meaning*. New York: St Martin's Press.

Thompson, M. (ed.) (1994) *Long Road to Freedom: The Advocate History of the Gay and Lesbian Movement*. New York: St Martin's Press.

Thompson, N. (1995) *Theory and Practice in Health and Social Welfare.* Buckingham: Open University Press.

Tiefer, L. (1995) *Sex is Not a Natural Act and Other Essays.* San Francisco: Westview.

Tinney, J. (1996) Why a Black Gay Church? Reprinted in M. Blasius and S. Phelan (eds) (1997) *We Are Everywhere: A Historical Sourcebook of Gay and Lesbian Politics.* London: Routledge.

Trades Unionists against Section 28 (TUAS28) (1989) *Out at Work: Campaigning for Lesbian and Gay Rights.* London: TUAS28 and City Limits.

Treichler, P. (1988) AIDS, gender and biomedical discourse: Current contests for meaning, in E. Fee and D. Fox (eds) *AIDS: The Burdens of History.* Berkeley, CA: University of California Press.

Trenchard, L. (1989) *Being Lesbian.* London: Gay Men's Press.

Trenchard, L. and Warren, H. (1984) *Something to Tell You.* London: London Gay Teenage Group.

Trippet, S. and Bain, J. (1993) Reasons American lesbians fail to seek traditional health care, in P.N. Stern (ed.) *Lesbian Health: What are the Issues?* London: Taylor & Francis.

Turner, B.S. (1995) *Medical Power and Social Knowledge.* London: Sage.

Vance, C. (ed.) (1981) *Pleasure and Danger: Exploring Female Sexuality.* London: Pandora.

Vance, C. (1988) Social construction theory: Problems in the history of sexuality, in C. Vance (ed.) *Which Homosexuality? Essays from the International Scientific Conference on Lesbian and Gay Studies.* London: Gay Men's Press.

van der Vliet, V. (1996) *The Politics of AIDS.* London: Bowerdeane.

VanEvery, J. (1996) Sinking into his arms . . . arms in his sink: Heterosexuality and Feminism Revisited, in L. Adkins and V. Merchant (eds) *Sexualizing the Social: Power and the Organization of Sexuality.* London: Macmillan/British Sociological Association.

Vida, G. (1978) *Our Right to Love: A Lesbian Resource Book.* Englewood Cliffs, NJ: Prentice Hall.

Vincent, C.-J. (1996) Lesbians, gay men and Christian fundamentalism, *Journal of Women Against Fundamentalism,* 8(1): 6–7.

Waldby, C. (1996) *AIDS and the Body Politic: Biomedicine and Sexual Difference.* London: Routledge.

Walker, A. and Parmar, P. (1993) *Warrior Marks: Female Genital Mutilation and the Sexual Blinding of Women.* London: Jonathan Cape.

War on Want (1996) *We've Declared War on Prejudice* (campaign booklet). London: War on Want.

Ware, V. (1992) *Beyond the Pale: White Women, Racism and History.* London: Verso.

Warland, B. (ed.) (1992) *InVersions: Writing by Dykes, Queers and Lesbians.* London: Open Letters.

Watney, S. (1987) *Policing Desire: Pornography, AIDS and the Media.* London: Methuen.

Webb, C. (1985) *Sexuality: Nursing and Health.* Chichester: John Wiley.

Weedon, C. (1987) *Feminist Practice and Poststructuralist Theory.* Oxford: Blackwell.

Weeks, J. (1985) *Sexualities and Its Discontents: Meanings, Myths and Modern Sexualities.* London: Routledge & Kegan Paul.

Weeks, J. (1986) *Sexuality.* London: Routledge.

Weeks, J. (1990) *Coming Out: Homosexual Politics in Britain from the Nineteenth Century to the Present,* revised edn. London: Quartet.

Weeks, J. (1991) *Against Nature: Essays on History, Sexuality and Identity.* London: Rivers Oram.

Weiner, G. and Arnot, M. (eds) (1987) *Gender Under Scrutiny: New Inquiries in Education.* Milton Keynes: Open University Press.

Wells, J. (1982) *A Herstory of Prostitution in Western Europe*. Berkeley, CA: Shameless Hussy Press.

Weston, K. (1993) Parenting in the age of AIDS, in A. Stein (ed.) *Sisters, Sexperts, Queers: Beyond the Lesbian Nation*. Harmondsworth: Penguin (Plume).

Weston, K. (1998) Families we choose, in P. Nardi and B. Schneider (eds) *Social Perspectives in Lesbian and Gay Studies: A Reader*. London: Routledge.

Whatley, M.H. (1992) Images of lesbians and gays in sexuality and health textbooks, *Journal of Homosexuality*, 22(3–4): 197–211.

Whisman, V. (1996) *Queer by Choice: Lesbians, Gay Men and the Politics of Identity*. London: Routledge.

White, E. (1982) *A Boy's Own Story*. London: Picador.

White, E. (1997) *The Farewell Symphony*. London: Chatto and Windus.

Whitehead, T. (1993) The voluntary sector: Five years on, in E. Carter and S. Watney (eds) *Taking Liberties: AIDS and Cultural Politics*. London: Serpent's Tail.

Whitlock, K. (1988) *Bridges of Respect: Creating Support for Lesbian and Gay Youth*. Philadelphia, PA: American Friends Service Committee.

Whyte, J., Deem, R., Kant, L. and Cruickshank, M. (eds) (1985) *Girl Friendly Schooling*. London: Methuen.

Wildeblood, P. (1955) *Against the Law*. Harmondsworth: Penguin.

Williams, F. (1989) *Social Policy: A Critical Introduction*. Cambridge: Polity.

Wilton, T. (1992) *Antibody Politic: AIDS and Society*. Cheltenham: New Clarion Press.

Wilton, T. (1993) Queer subjects: Lesbians, heterosexual women and the academy, in M. Kennedy, C. Lubelska and V. Walsh (eds) *Making Connections: Women's Studies, Women's Movements, Women's Lives*. London: Taylor & Francis.

Wilton, T. (1995) *Lesbian Studies: Setting an Agenda*. London: Routledge.

Wilton, T. (1996) *Finger-Licking Good: The Ins and Outs of Lesbian Sex*. London: Cassell.

Wilton, T. (1997a) *En/Gendering AIDS: Deconstructing Sex, Texts and Epidemic*. London: Sage.

Wilton, T. (1997b) *Good For You: A Handbook on Lesbian Health and Wellbeing*. London: Cassell.

Wilton, T. (1998) Gender, sexuality and healthcare: improving services, in L. Doyal (ed.) *Women and Health Services*. Buckingham: Open University Press.

Wilton, T. (1999a) Going through the change, *Diva*, April: 34–5.

Wilton, T. (1999b) *Second Best Value: Lesbian, Gay and Bisexual Life in Bristol*. Bristol: Lesbian, Gay and Bisexual Forum.

Wilton, T. and Hall, C. (1998) Healthcare experiences of lesbians, gay men and bisexuals in the Bristol area. Unpublished summary of research in progress, Faculty of Health and Social Care, University of the West of England.

Wittig, M. (1992) *The Straight Mind and Other Essays*. Hemel Hempstead: Harvester Wheatsheaf.

World Health Organization (WHO) (1992) *School Health Education to Prevent AIDS and Sexually Transmitted Diseases*. Geneva: WHO and UNESCO.

World Health Organization (WHO) (1995) *Facing the Challenges of HIV, AIDS, STDs: A Gender-based Response*. Geneva: Royal Tropical Institute, South Africa AIDS Information Dissemination Service and World Health Organization Global Programme on AIDS.

Wrench, N. (1998) Stop badgering the buggers, *Gay Times*, May: 11–12.

Ziegler, P. (1979) *The Black Death*. Stroud: Sutton.

Zita, J. (1992) The male lesbian and the postmodernist body, in C. Card (ed.) *Hypatia*, 7(4) (special issue: Lesbian Philosophy): 106–27.

index